Understanding and Treating
Hot Flashes in Menopause
with Chinese Medicine

UNDERSTANDING AND TREATING HOT FLASHES IN MENOPAUSE WITH CHINESE MEDICINE

BRIAN GROSAM, PhD, LAc

Foreword by Yubin Lu, PhD, LAc

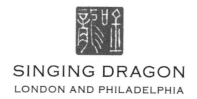

SINGING DRAGON

LONDON AND PHILADELPHIA

First published in Great Britain in 2022 by Singing Dragon,
an imprint of Jessica Kingsley Publishers
An Hachette Company

1

Copyright © Dr. Brian Grosam 2022
Foreword copyright © Dr. Yubin Lu 2022

Front cover image source: Shutterstock®.

The information contained in this book is not intended to replace the services of trained medical professionals or to be a substitute for medical advice. The complementary therapy described in this book may not be suitable for everyone to follow. You are advised to consult a doctor before embarking on any complementary therapy program and on any matters relating to your health, and in particular on any matters that may require diagnosis or medical attention.

A CIP catalogue record for this title is available from the
British Library and the Library of Congress

ISBN 978 1 78775 538 3
eISBN 978 1 78775 539 0

Printed and bound by CPI Group (UK) Ltd, Croydon, CR0 4YY

Jessica Kingsley Publishers' policy is to use papers that are natural, renewable and recyclable products and made from wood grown in sustainable forests. The logging and manufacturing processes are expected to conform to the environmental regulations of the country of origin.

Jessica Kingsley Publishers
Carmelite House
50 Victoria Embankment
London EC4Y 0DZ

www.singingdragon.com

*This book is dedicated to
my mom and dad.*

Contents

Foreword by Yubin Lu, PhD, LAc. 11

Acknowledgments 15

Preface. 17

1. Hot Flashes—Chinese-Medicine Theory 21
   The Hot-Flash Environment   21
   Huangdi Neijing Suwen—Female Years of Seven   27
   Chao Re—Tides of Heat   31
   Heat and Fire—The Hot Flash   34
   Aspects of Qi   40
   Aspects of Blood   47
   Aspects of Yin and Yang   53
   Wei Qi   60

2. Hot Flashes—Zangfu Organ Theory 63
   Zangfu Organ Associations   63
   The Kidney—The Foundation   64
   The Kidney and the Heart   65
   The Heart—The Monarch   66
   The Kidney and the Liver   67
   The Kidney and the Spleen and Stomach   68
   The Kidney and the Lung   69
   The Kidney and the Lower Jiao   70
   The Kidney and the Brain   70
   Conclusion   71

3. Hot Flashes—Classical Chinese-Medicine Theory 73

Classical Chinese Medicine   73

Shang Han Lun   74

Nan Jing   79

Pi Wei Lun   84

The Fire Spirit School   88

Fu Qing Zhu Gynecology   91

4. Hot Flashes—Chinese Medicine Meets Western Medicine . . .   99

Introduction—The Hot Flash   99

Menopausal Transition   99

Chinese-Medicine Pathophysiology   100

Thermoregulation   102

HPO Axis   102

Hormones   105

Does Estrogen Deprivation Alone Cause Hot Flashes?   108

Reproductive Aging   112

Western-Medicine Treatment Approaches   114

Predisposed Menopause and Artificial Menopause   118

Conclusion   120

5. Hot Flashes—Chinese-Medicine Diagnosis 121

Introduction   121

Effective Hot-Flash Diagnosis   122

The Congenital and Acquired Constitutions   123

The Five Zang—Lifestyle Habits   125

Diagnosing Hot-Flash Patterns   128

Axis, Trajectories, and Triads   133

Frequency, Severity, and Duration   137

Hot Flashes and the Time of Day   142

Respiration—Balance of the Lung and Kidney   150

Temperature and Tolerance   154

Patient Initial Health Intake   156

Surgically Induced Hot Flashes   185

Pharmaceuticals-Induced Hot Flashes   186

6. Treating Hot Flashes with Acupuncture 195

Introduction 195

Treatment Approaches to Hot Flashes 196

Acupuncture Hypersensitivity and Needling Techniques 204

Traditional Hot-Flash Acupuncture Prescriptions 212

Clinical Research 217

Quantity and Frequency of Treatments 225

Treatment Schedule 228

Clinical Hot-Flash Point Prescriptions 229

Hot-Flash Acupuncture Modifications 243

Back Acupuncture Treatments 259

Auricular Acupuncture 261

Acupuncture and Hot Flashes Scientific Research 263

7. Treating Hot Flashes with Chinese Herbal Medicine 269

Treatment Principles 269

Hot-Flash Herbal Formulas 270

Traditional Tidal Heat Effusion Herbal Formulas 276

Excess Heat and Fire Prescriptions 278

Repletion and Stagnation Prescriptions 286

Qi and Blood Deficiency Prescriptions 297

Yin Deficiency Prescriptions 302

Yang Deficiency Prescriptions 308

Calming the Spirit Prescriptions 310

References. 317

Further Reading 321

About the Author 323

Index 325

Foreword

Removing the Veil Covering the Hot Flash

Dr. Grosam has been exploring the mechanisms and clinical treatments of menopausal transition ever since he chose the effects of acupuncture in treating hot flashes as the topic for his dissertation years ago. I have wondered how far he could go with this topic, since hot flashes are often considered a simple symptom in the clinic. Reading his book, I was surprised and pleased. I applaud him for this excellent work.

For the first time in Chinese-medicine history, the hot flash is discussed extensively, with many confusions clarified. Most practitioners think it is kidney yin deficiency that causes the hot flash, a result of failure of deficient yin to restrict yang. But in many cases, treatment based on this belief does not work as well as would be expected. There must be something missing in understanding the mechanisms of the hot flash. The extensive discussion in this book unveils the real face of the hot flash and makes it possible to understand the underlying environment of the symptom and thus provide more effective treatments for patients.

First, Dr. Grosam puts forward the idea that hot flashes are closely related to the loss of blood in females due to the monthly menstrual cycle. By menopause, blood is deficient, yang will not be held, and it floats upwards to generate the hot flash. The model adopted in this book, showing how yang can float when blood is lost, is brilliant. One conclusion—tonifying blood plays an important role in the treatment of hot flashes.

Second, this book provides a detailed discussion on some tough theoretical problems related to the hot flash, such as yin fire, tidal fever, heat due to qi deficiency, the relationship of water and fire, the relationship of sovereign fire and ministerial fire, etc., which are all critical in explaining the mechanisms of hot flashes.

Using the taijitu narrative, this book clearly discusses how yin and yang of the heart and kidney change and how that gives rise to hot flashes. The idea that yin has to follow yang to ascend and yang has to follow yin to descend is extremely important. The relationship between the heart fire and kidney water is an excellent highlight in the explanation of the mechanism of the hot flash.

Dr. Grosam also clarifies how hot flashes can result from excess heat or fire in the heart, liver, or yangming fu organs. I find another theory presented in this book to be very important. It describes the role of qi deficiency and qi stagnation. Stagnation produces heat. Qi deficiency can contribute to the development of hot flashes due to its failure to promote movement.

Third, this book clearly summarizes the differential diagnosis of many types of hot flashes and the corresponding acupuncture and herbal treatments for these hot flashes. After reading the book, readers will have a much clearer understanding of the pathogenesis, diagnosis, and treatments of hot flashes. This will lead to more effective treatments for hot-flash patients from Chinese-medicine practitioners.

Any theoretical hypothesis must be tested by clinical practice. Dr. Li Dongyuan had to face the theoretical frustration when he was treating fever with qi tonics, since qi belongs to yang and qi deficiency should cause more cold conditions than heat in light of yinyang theory. Although doctors of later generations have been trying to find a clear answer to this issue, no one can deny that the treatment of tonifying qi to clear heat works well in the clinic when applied correctly. As his basic focus in the past ten years, Dr. Grosam has treated many patients with hot flashes and compared the effectiveness of the different treatments based on different theories. There is no doubt that understanding the mechanism of the hot flash from multiple perspectives and treating hot flashes based on the different mechanisms is much more effective than just nourishing kidney yin and clearing heat or purging fire.

It is easy to find a leaf in a big tree but hard to find the tree in a leaf. Without years of clinical and theoretical study of hot flashes,

Dr. Grosam could not have written this book. If more Chinese-medicine practitioners follow this path in their practice and research, there will be more rapid progress in the development of Chinese medicine. I hope a Chinese-language version of this book will be accessible to the Chinese-medicine practitioners in China soon.

Yubin Lu, PhD, LAc

Acknowledgments

I would first and foremost like to thank my mentor and friend, Dr. Yubin Lu, a true Chinese-medicine scholar and herbal master. You have instilled in me your mastery of Chinese-medicine theory, which has served as the foundation of my clinical practice and knowledge of our medicine. You taught me that Chinese medicine is a long journey and to be patient, trust myself, and grow with time.

Thank you, Dr. Wen Jiang, my acupuncture guru and dear friend. Thank you for your kind heart and generous support. You were always there every time I asked for and needed it. I honor you for being true to our acupuncture lineage.

A special thank you to my uncle, James Hartmann, my surrogate father and male role model. I am truly blessed to have you in my life. Thank you for editing my book. This book would not have been possible or come to fruition without your help. I love you.

Thank you to Dr. Qihua Shan and Dr. Fudong Wu for accepting me into your acupuncture lineage and mentoring me through my PhD studies. You are my acupuncture parents and mentors. Dr. Shan, in clinic you provided the understanding that acupuncture is about accuracy, repetition, patience, concentration, continual learning, and honing one's clinical skills. I am forever grateful.

A special thank you to Juan Liu, my Chinese language teacher. First, you helped my family with finding the best medical care while living in China. Your compassion helped us through some potential life-threatening situations. Second, you bestowed upon me the precious gift of Chinese language. With this knowledge, I am able to understand

Chinese medicine at a deeper level. I truly cherish the time we spent together.

To my dear friends Julie McCormick and Joi Thomas—thank you! You always believed in me even when I didn't. I cherish your everlasting encouragement, support, and optimism. You are my tribe and family.

Thank you to my fellow colleagues, scholars of Chinese medicine, past students, peers, and, most of all, patients. I've learned so much from all of you. I'd be half the practitioner without you.

A sincere thank you to Claire Wilson, Claire Robinson, Maddy Budd, and the rest of the Singing Dragon team for all of your diligence and hard work helping make my book a reality. I'm deeply indebted.

I bow my head with the greatest respect to the great Chinese-medicine masters and practitioners of the past. Thank you for your wisdom and guidance. I feel your presence deep within my shen. I am honored to have learned from your knowledge and experience.

The deepest thank you goes to my family. To my wife, Pamela, thank you for everything! The love and support, patience, encouragement, and, above all, introducing me to Chinese medicine all those years ago. You are my inspiration. You are the true master of qi and goddess of energy. I am always learning from your energy and love. You are too good to be true! Last, but not least, thank you to my two sons Maxwell and Jaxon. You are my joy and inspiration. May you find yourselves in this lifetime and may your hearts be filled with love.

Brian Grosam, PhD, LAc
古龙

Preface

"Something wonderful is about to happen to you."

I received this message via fortune cookie while celebrating our seventh wedding anniversary immediately after the opportunity to study acupuncture and Chinese medicine was presented to me. I carried this fortune in my wallet every day until I graduated with my PhD in acupuncture eight years later. Now framed, the fortune adorns our clinic waiting room wall to greet everyone who enters our healing space.

This fortune represents my calling to Chinese medicine. I always say that the medicine chose me. It was a long, strange path. My undergraduate degree is in art. I studied at the American Academy of Acupuncture and Oriental Medicine (AAAOM) in Minnesota and then uprooted my wife and two sons, selling everything we had, to live and study in Jinan, China for three years from 2006 to 2009. There was no organized timeline or map for this journey!

I am reminded every day of the power and beauty of our medicine. It is so much more than solving health issues, eliminating symptoms, and curing ailments. It is about changing the trajectories of people's lives towards health and positivity. When people experience Chinese medicine, they can begin a new journey and my fortune expands—something wonderful happens to them, too!

My experience of researching and doing the clinical trials on treating menopausal transition with acupuncture for my dissertation left me with the understanding that my work was not completed—in fact, it had only just begun. My time as a formal student ended, but my learning just entered a new phase. I had so many new questions that needed answers. I realize now that those eight years of learning and training as a PhD candidate were merely establishing a foundation of knowledge upon which a lifetime of learning would be built. My professor, Dr. Yubin Lu, once told me that the goal of the doctoral process is to condition you to learn and think on your own so that your real growth as a doctor can begin.

Of all the symptoms women experience during menopausal transition, the hot flash is the one they most often speak about and seek treatment for. It is remarkable that a subject can have such a profound influence on women's lives and yet have such scattered and incomplete medical references.

Women came to me seeking support and treatment and I gave them the best I could. I continued to do research and developed and tested new theories. The more I learned through my practice, the more I needed to know. When I found there was no book that could provide the systematic approach to help women manage this medical challenge I needed, the answer became obvious. I would have to write it myself! With that understanding, I gathered my courage and contacted Claire Wilson at Singing Dragon to accept her offer to write this book.

When I began writing, it was clear I needed to write from my head and my heart and include my own personal journey and clinical experience pertinent to hot flashes. This book is an attempt to bring together my experience over ten years of clinical practice… my clinical notes, treatment approaches, medical theories, and general ideas on hot flashes… and to summarize them in a way that will help other practitioners improve their medical support for women.

Trying to organize the overlap of theories upon theories, each one blending into the others, some contradicting and some complementing each other, was like ironing out a cobweb. Truthfully, there were times I thought I could never sort it out, let alone organize it into a finished and cohesive document. The insight that helped me complete this project was the realization that I would not be able to describe every theory and every pattern involved in the hot-flash environment—and that I didn't have to! I realized I was not writing the last book on this topic—I was creating one link in a chain of developing knowledge.

I am very proud of this book. I don't consider myself a very strong writer nor am I a scholarly man, but I have been thinking about hot flashes and treating women for a long time. There are so many underlying dynamics going on in the female body during menopausal transition; it is not reasonable to hope to encompass all of the knowledge and theories in a single book. What is possible is to create a common understanding upon which future learning can be built.

My hope is that individuals who read this book will gain deeper understanding of the unique and beautiful energetic changes happening within every woman. The phoenix on the cover symbolizes the magical yin and yang, fire and water dynamic occurring during menopausal transition. But more importantly, it represents a spiritual *and societal* change in all women—a rebirth of the physical, emotional, and spiritual.

This book is intended as a resource that will help practitioners develop a core understanding of the hot-flash environment through the traditions of Chinese medicine. If it serves its purpose, it will encourage more effective treatment for women now and research that will lead to better understanding and improved treatments in the future.

Chapter 1

Hot Flashes—Chinese-Medicine Theory

The Hot-Flash Environment

Hot flashes are a common symptom for women during perimenopause and menopausal transition, the years leading up to, during, and following menopause. In Western medicine, hot flashes are considered the direct effect of a drop in estrogen from the naturally occurring ovarian reserve decline, thus affecting the hypothalamic-pituitary-ovarian (HPO) axis. This creates an environment in the hypothalamus that disrupts thermoregulation, its ability to control body temperature. The parameters of control are narrowed, meaning that the hypothalamus has less ability to control temperature and leaving it easily susceptible to stimulation. Such stimulation can come from a multitude of lifestyle stimuli. Stimulation is thought to disrupt neurotransmitters in the brain, causing a cascade of responses leading to hypothalamus thermoregulation disruption and hot flashes.

The Western medical community widely accepts the conclusion that hot flashes are the direct result of the decline of ovarian estrogen, which is oftentimes easily treatable in the Western medical clinics with hormone therapies (HTs) and more current treatments to regulate neurotransmitters, such as increasing serotonin levels or normalizing norepinephrine levels with selective serotonin-reuptake inhibitors (SSRIs) and serotonin norepinephrine-reuptake inhibitors (SNRIs). These pharmaceuticals can sometimes be a viable short-term option to treat severe or intractable hot flashes, but they also carry potential severe health risks. This generates the need for safe and effective alternatives to pharmaceutical treatments like acupuncture and Chinese herbal medicine. My main objectives are to gain a better understanding of the hot-flash physiology and pathomechanisms from the Chinese medical perspective, to understand it alongside the current Western medicine hot-flash framework, and to enhance our diagnosis skills and treatment efficacy.

Chinese medicine takes a holistic approach to understanding and treating the body with its nature-oriented physiological understandings of qi (energy), blood (nutrition), yin and yang, five-phase, zangfu (internal) organs, jing (essence), shen (spirit), and the channel (meridian) system, which connects every tissue in the body. One of these factors working independently or several working simultaneously may be and are often involved in the creation of what I call "the hot-flash environment."

The primary question we need to explore when investigating the hot-flash environment is: "Which pieces of the above-mentioned concepts are imbalanced or not functioning correctly?" That is a key goal of our discussion: to peer through the multiple conceptual layers Chinese medicine utilizes, to truly comprehend what is at the root, creating the hot flash. We need to think and look beyond the Western medicine idea of thermoregulation and the Chinese-medicine concept of "yin deficiency heat." After all, the situational imbalance and cause of a hot flash can oftentimes be a complex cascade or series of events, which can make it difficult to diagnose and treat.

In the acupuncture clinic, it is far too easy to treat hot flashes by naively nourishing yin to quell the heat or merely trying to clear a pathogenic fire. It may work sometimes, but if you treat hot flashes, sooner or later you'll end up scratching your head, wondering why those treatments aren't working. To truly be able to help difficult hot-flash cases, we must see and understand how the hot flash is presenting as a symptom by examining and understanding the internal environment.

There are many perspectives to the hot-flash environment and many of our Chinese-medicine theories overlap and blend into one another, which can sometimes make analysis unclear and confusing. The body is a vast ocean of energy and substance. In Chinese medicine, we think in terms of qi, blood, yinyang, jing (essence), and shen (spirit). Together, they function along a multitude of intertwining currents. These currents are a combination of gravitational trajectories, ebbing and flowing tides, axis rotations, pendulums, bellows, electrical circuits, fluid evaporation and precipitation, and irrigation systems. They all work in unison at various strengths and timing for the sole purpose of supporting an optimal living environment. It is necessary for these currents of energy and substance to naturally change in strength and function over time and with age to support growth, health, and longevity. By discussing each of these concepts, we can understand the many functional possibilities that take place in order to create the hot-flash environment. When the clinician can thoroughly comprehend these underlying functional possibilities, one can then accurately diagnose the source of the hot flashes and effectively administer medical treatment to the patient.

Bursts of Qi

Feelings of waves of heat from within the body can happen at any age in both men and women and can be the result of numerous issues relating to digestion, emotional issues, qi and blood imbalances, or exposure to external pathogenic factors. Conversely, hot flashes are a symptom stemming from a completely different source, specific to women, and manifest during the times of perimenopause, menopausal transition, and post-menopause. Since they are of a unique nature, they must be looked at, diagnosed, and treated differently in order for the practitioner to be successful.

At the most basic level, the hot flash is a burst of qi from within rising to the surface and exiting the body. Hot flashes are a series of bursts of qi that are triggered and released by the hot-flash environment, and to fully understand them, we need to investigate the various currents and individual systems of the natural fire sources, the ebb and flow of qi and blood, the balance of yin and yang, and the communication of the zangfu organs. When there are disruptions to this large interactive system, problems arise, such as deficiencies, excesses, and stagnations, which in turn give rise to bursts of qi and symptoms of heat.

But what causes these bursts? It is my belief that hot flash originates in the blood. After decades of monthly menstrual cycles, it is easy to understand that the blood would be a component. It takes a great deal of energy to release and rebuild blood month after month. There are many ways the blood can fall into dysfunction or deficiency scenarios. The second important aspect is the balance of yin and yang. The yin has its relationship to nutrition and the blood, while the yang has its relationship to physiological function and qi. Our lifestyle habits can have an enormous impact on their overall balance, leading to relative excesses and deficiencies. Over time, these imbalances of yin and yang can trigger and set into motion the pieces that generate the hot-flash environment. Finally, various stagnations throughout the body, including the channel and zangfu organ systems, can produce or accentuate the hot flash. Stagnations throughout the body have many internal and external environmental causes.

It is probable there will be several simultaneous issues coming together to create the hot-flash environment, including deficiencies, excesses, and stagnations. One must understand the individual patient's hot-flash environment and the complexities of her internal environment to effectively diagnose and treat.

Why Do Some Women Experience Hot Flashes While Others Do Not?

I believe that there are a number of reasons why some women do not experience hot flashes, involving their genetics, history of illnesses, and lifestyle habits. In Chinese medicine, these categories are considered either the "pre-heaven" or "post-heaven" qi, meaning there are some traits we are born with and are naturally inclined to that were decided before we were born, and other traits we can attribute to our health history and our choices in life, like our dietary decisions, exercise habits, mental-emotional status, activity, sleep patterns, and overall spiritual fulfillment.

Over the first four to five decades of a woman's life, the two categories will slowly ebb, flow, intertwine, and develop a unique internal environment and personal body chemistry that constitutes her hot-flash environment. What we will discuss in this book is exactly how the hot-flash environment comes into formation.

Ten-Women Scenario

Consider a group of ten women who are experiencing hot flashes. It is probable that even though all are going through menopausal transition, with a natural decline of ovarian estrogen, their individual diagnoses will have considerable differences.

Chinese medicine takes age into consideration and it's presumable that most women will have a decline in jing (essence). The jing really means the kidney essence, which includes both kidney yin and kidney yang qi. This is the natural physiological piece; the kidney essence naturally declines with age in all species.

If these were the only physiological issues involved and are universal in all women, the natural conclusion at this point from both the Western and Chinese medical points of view would be that every woman would experience hot flashes. Yet hot flashes are not universal. There must be other factors involved in the creation of the hot-flash environment.

Every woman is unique in her genetic makeup, lifestyle habits and choices, history of illnesses, and environmental factors, and this combination will shape her menopausal transition. Our diets, nutrition, and hydration have an impact on our body. Impacts like stress and other emotional strife, exposure to artificial environments, movement and activity, pharmaceuticals, and so on all play roles. What is ultimately taking place inside our body in today's society has everything to do with how we age, function, and present with symptoms.

With the sharp increase in hot-flash symptoms in the modern era, especially in highly developed industrialized nations, we need to look closely at the main lifestyle and societal changes from the past to the present. It is a viable conclusion that hot flashes are a natural aging side effect to estrogen decline but are more prominent today due to the above-mentioned lifestyle issues and inherited genetic makeup. This is the key concept driving many clinical questions regarding hot flashes, including frequency, duration, and severity. The clinician must consider the patient's internal physiological environment and the roles that genetics and lifestyle habits play in the patient's situation.

Returning to our group of ten women… the absence or presence and severity of hot flashes will be vastly different from one woman to the next. The adept practitioner can guide women in analyzing the ways in which their environment and personal choices may be affecting their hot-flash environments. Factors such as food triggers, lack of hydration, fatigue, insomnia, overworking, a lack of exercise, or high stress may ignite the hot-flash environment. Many women, in fact, can self-treat and ameliorate hot flashes over time by modifying their lifestyle habits. Chinese medicine has always incorporated this approach, and more recently it is gaining acceptance in Western medicine as well.

Ultimately, hot flashes are the end-product symptom of the decline of essence, an internal imbalance or miscommunication within the body, and lifestyle stimuli. The Chinese internal medical terrain is a vast and detailed map that often separates the mediocre from the masterful practitioner. Understanding and observing the relationship between qi and blood, the excesses and deficiencies of yin and yang, and the imbalances of the zangfu organs is the key to revealing these imbalances and miscommunications in each patient.

Every hot flash, then, should be considered a symptom stemming from the individual's unique medical terrain. Each of the ten women in our group will have a unique hot-flash environment, different from her counterparts. The holistic approach of Chinese medicine helps decide the most appropriate treatment that is correctly targeted for the individual patient and not merely a "treat-all" approach. In the case of the hot-flash environment, the practitioner's role is to identify each patient's unique reality and to employ appropriate strategies to address causes as well as symptoms.

The goal of this book is to detail the physiological circumstances of deficiencies, excesses, and stagnations that combine to generate internal bursts of qi and heat and how these translate into the hot flash. Taking into account that the hot-flash environment is a conglomerate of a natural phenomenon, pathogenic factors, symptoms from the internal environment, and the overall vitality of the individual, our discussion will break these topics down into individual components.

The central focus is on the balance of yin and yang in terms of qi and blood, zangfu organs, the channel system, and the neuro-endocrine system. Understanding the yin and yang balance can shed light on the mechanisms behind hot flashes and how we can treat them effectively. Chinese medical practitioners will understand that internal imbalances and disruptions are all intertwined: one causes the next, and one consumes the other, and one flows into the new.

We will discuss the hot flash itself in detail as a symptom and as an entity. From a Chinese-medicine theoretical perspective, we will look at hot flashes from many angles to understand the possibilities of their origin, including the yinyang cycle, the pathology of heat, and the zangfu organ system. We will also utilize the classical Chinese medical texts to support our newly found understandings. Based on this integrated knowledge, we will discuss clinical treatment approaches including diagnosis, treatment principles, and the roles acupuncture, herbal-medicine formulas, and lifestyle changes can play in treatment.

Huangdi Neijing Suwen—Female Years of Seven

There are few classical medical entries, in Eastern or Western medicine, that discuss in detail or represent a theoretical basis that describes the decline of a woman's ovarian reserve and the drop of estrogen, leading to the hot flash and other menopausal symptoms. Though there are many references to age and the cessation of menstruation, there is little discussion of hot flashes, which leaves us to rely on our interpretation of the classics and apply it to the modern era. One famous reference in Chinese medicine, written more than 2000 years ago, that gives us plenty of clues and a theoretical foundation to base further theories and understandings upon is found in the first chapter of the *Huangdi Neijing Suwen*. You may be familiar with this quotation from your study of Chinese medicine:

> In a female, at the age of seven, the qi of the kidneys abounds. The [first] teeth are substituted and the hair grows long. With two times seven, the heaven *gui* arrives, the controlling vessel is passable and the great thoroughfare vessel abounds [with qi]. The monthly affair

moves down in due time and, hence, [a woman] may have children. With three times seven, the qi of the kidneys has reached its normal level. Hence, the wisdom teeth emerge and [females] grow to their full size. With four times seven, the sinews and bones are firm and the hair has grown to its full extent. The body and the limbs are in a state of abundance and strength. With five times seven, the yang brilliance vessel weakens; the face begins to dry out; the hair begins to fall off. With six times seven, the three yang vessels weaken {in the upper sections}. The face is parched, the hair begins to turn white. With seven times seven, the controlling vessel is depleted and the great thoroughfare vessel is weak and [its contents are] diminished. The heaven *gui* is exhausted. The way of the earth is impassable. Hence, the physical appearance is spoilt and [a woman can] no [longer] have children. (Unschuld and Tessenow 2011, pp.36–39)

This passage presents a classic Chinese-medicine perspective on the physical maturation of women in seven-year increments and it forms the gynecological backdrop for the menstrual cycle, fertility, and menopause.

In terms of hot flashes however, it really doesn't give us a direct indication as to the reasoning or cause behind them. Or does it? This entry refers to the root "change" in the body system without giving us a real "cause." If we utilize our Chinese-medicine knowledge and critical thinking, we can use this writing as a foundation and begin to build a theory for a deeper understanding of the hot flash. This quotation gives us much Chinese gynecological medical theory and highlights the general rising and falling of hormone levels within the female body and how the conception age comes to fruition at menarche and declines at menopause.

Let's begin by examining the increment ages of 14, 21, and 28. Here we find out that the tiangui (heavenly dew) arrives and the chong and ren vessels fill up and flow with blood. Tiangui is another term for the menstrual blood, and it originates from the kidney essence (yin). This indicates that the hormones and uterus have been established for the menstrual cycle and fertility. Gradually, over the next seven years to the age of 21, the kidney essence becomes the solid foundation for the zangfu organs and the woman's body becomes strong and healthy. By age 28, the text indicates that a woman reaches her peak of vitality and strength.

The *Neijing* entry finally becomes directly relevant to our hot-flash discussion with its description of age 35. It describes a shift in the strength of qi and the decline of the yangming channels that we know are rich in qi and blood. The yangming are the stomach and the large intestine channels. They are the two that provide the body with energy and strength and the zangfu organs with qi and blood. The gradually declining yangming, as we see, lose their strength to bring nourishment to the tissues, and the first signs of aging present as dryness in the face and hair. In understanding this process, we can be observant of these changes in the clinical setting.

By age 42, the yang qi has already reached its peak of energy and now begins its decline. The true yang energy of the body (mingmen or life gate) represents vitality, strength throughout the zangfu organ system, and the ability to conceive a child. This coincides with current data and the difficulty for women to conceive past this age. The importance of the concept of yang qi decline is the effect it has on the mingmen and the kidney as the source of our root yang fire. It also supports our understanding that when we pass age 42, women (and men) begin to experience this gradual weakening of the kidney essence, thereby the yin and yang qi of the kidney are liable to fall out of equilibrium. The human body is an integral whole, so this deficiency of the kidney will inevitably affect the other zangfu organs, leading to disequilibrium in the functioning of the entire zangfu system and giving rise to a series of common Chinese medical kidney deficiency symptoms. But to clarify... though the kidney has reached its peak and begins its gradual decline, and this has an important influence on overall health, the kidney is not the root cause of menopausal-transition symptoms or hot flashes.

The following is commentary from this *Neijing* passage. I find it a particularly important key to understanding the root cause of the hot flash. "With six times seven, the three yang vessels weaken {in the upper sections}." Commentary: "The reason for their weakness lies in the nature of females. They have a surplus of qi and a deficiency of blood, because [the latter] is frequently drained by the way of menstruation" (Unschuld and Tessenow 2011, pp.38–39).

So how does this "weakness" potentially create an environment in which a woman's body begins to generate a tide of consistent heat waves that radiate upwards and outwards? The answer is clear: There is a deficiency of blood and an abundance of qi. This is due to the slow and progressive loss of blood via decades of a monthly menstrual cycle. A woman's blood surplus is slowly diminished one month at a time, creating an imbalance of yin (blood) and yang (qi), creating an environment of qi abundance. This abundance of qi has the potential to cycle abnormally—faster, slower, and at irregular times… or bursts of qi. This is a yin and yang and a water and fire concept. When the blood is exhausted, there is only an abundance of qi left over. Qi here is heat and this heat represents hot flashes. The root cause then is blood deficiency.

I find the close proximity of age 49 to the time of menopause in our modern times, a median age of 51.3, to be quite interesting to say the least. Our reference says that by age 49, the tiangui has been exhausted—meaning a woman's ovarian reserve is completely depleted and there is an inevitable decline of hormone levels. The tiangui is exhausted, the ren and chong vessels are empty and not flowing, and the liver is no longer filled with blood. This natural physiological change can no longer support the natural functioning of menstruation and conception.

What can we conclude from this *Neijing* passage and commentary regarding the root cause of the hot flash?

It has always been a Chinese-medicine understanding that the decline of kidney essence (yin and yang qi) is part of the natural aging process and menopause around age 49 is the result. It has also been a general consensual understanding that the imbalance of kidney yin and yang qi eventually disrupts the overall yin and yang imbalance throughout the zangfu organs. In particular, this creates a water/fire imbalance between the kidney and heart. This results in a natural kidney (water) deficiency and a heart (fire) excess, leading to the conclusion that the hot flash is synonymous to heart fire.

Although I agree with the general theory of the kidney decline and also that the heart, and disruption to the heart, can be found at the center of the hot-flash environment, I do not believe this gives us a one-size-fits-all diagnosis. While these are fundamental truths, they are only a small portion of a much larger picture that we need to see to understand hot flashes.

The most vital takeaway from this *Neijing* passage is the gradual decline of the blood. Blood is nourishing, it is warming and cooling, and it balances the qi. There is also a harmony of yin and yang within the blood itself. When the blood is disrupted from excess, deficiency, heat, cold, stagnation, etc., the yin and yang within and throughout the body is disrupted as well. Understanding this and the vital role blood plays in menopause and in the creation of the hot-flash environment is crucial in treating hot flashes.

Chao Re—Tides of Heat

Let's start this discussion by taking a look into what the Chinese call "chao re." The two characters 潮热 chao re mean "hot flash" or "tidal heat effusion" and in Chinese medicine beautifully illustrate the internal yin and yang, water and fire interaction that engenders the hot-flash environment.

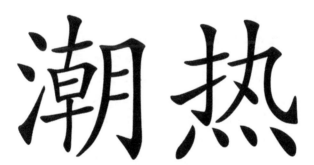

FIGURE 1.1: CHAO RE—CHINESE CHARACTERS

In Chinese medicine, chao re is described as: "Heat effusion, sometimes only felt subjectively, occurring at regular intervals, usually in the afternoon or evening" (Wiseman and Ye 1998, p.613). This definition is accurate, as hot flashes are basically the general feelings of heat manifesting from within the body that rush outwards to the skin surface at a regular ebb and flow or tidal intervals.

But even though the term chao re is interchangeable and commonly used to denote hot flashes in the medical community, the description of chao re in classical Chinese medicine carries a much broader definition and can oftentimes explain several completely different types of heat issues unrelated to the menopausal-transition hot flash. Understanding the term chao re in greater detail, including its meaning and classical medical significance, sets the foundation for our entire discussion.

The first recorded use of chao re can be found in the Chinese medical text *Shang Han Lun*. Chao re is used 24 times in this book and is generally used to describe internal heat repletion and stagnation patterns, which will be discussed later in Chapter 3. It is interesting to note that though hot flashes are sometimes described as being due to heat repletion and stagnation patterns, they are more commonly associated with deficiency issues of yin, yang, blood, essence, etc. As I began my studies into the effects of acupuncture and herbal medicine on treating hot flashes, I was sometimes confused by this dual use of terminology. With time and experience, I came to the understanding that the term chao re can represent hot flashes as a symptom, but it doesn't necessarily refer to the underlying physiological conditions causing them.

There are five causes or classifications of tidal heat effusion in classical Chinese medicine including: yin deficiency and blood depletion; yangming excess; spleen and stomach qi deficiency; damp-evil obstruction; blood stasis. In later chapters, we will take a closer look at how these patterns are viewed in different classical Chinese medical texts and discuss in detail the many probable and theoretical causes of hot flashes. The discussion will mainly focus on understanding the creation and generation of heat or fire within the body. But for now, let's break down the chao re characters and extract a few clues.

Chao 潮: The first character means "tide"… the coming and going, like the tides of the sea, much like hot flashes come and go in intervals, like waves. Chao 潮 should not be confused with another Chinese medical character chao 炒, which means to prepare food or herbs by "stir-frying" methods. The confusion can easily be misleading to a

Chinese medical practitioner by giving the idea of something being cooked like the yin within the body with a yang result of that being the release of heat. It does narrowly make some sense in describing how a yin deficiency can result in yang excess, but generally, a pathogenic heat inside cooking and drying up yin does not commonly cause menopausal-transition hot flashes.

"Chao" 潮 translates as "tide," "flow," "damp," or "wet." The character can be broken into two parts: The radical for water (shui) 水 is represented on the left by three dots, while the "chao" (zhao) character 朝 is represented on the right, which gives us the phonetic and can be interpreted to mean "dawn" or "morning." We can further break down the "chao" character 朝 into two parts: The cart or vehicle "che" character represented on the left, which is made up from the sun character centered between two plants, and the moon "yue" 月 is represented on the right.

This gives us an interesting look into the term "chao" in terms of yin and yang. Making use of the sun and moon alongside water highlights the rhythmic intervals of the tide. Chao is water (yin) and represents rhythm and the control or balance of the fire (yang) within the body or "re" 热. Chao also represents water (yin) in the form of sweat that often coincides with hot flashes, which is fire (yang).

Re 热 (熱): The second character means "heat" and is a bit more self-explanatory and straightforward. Hot flashes are the feeling of heat manifesting from within the body. "Re" can also mean enthusiasm, lively, excitement, or joy. I find this quite interesting because in Chinese medicine, joy is the emotion attributed to the heart. The heart, which is yang, also plays an integral role in the balance of hot flashes. Along with the kidney, which is yin, the heart and kidney control the ebb and flow of fire and water throughout the body. Hot flashes are sometimes a result of the imbalance of these two organs.

The character "re" 热 can be first broken down into the upper and lower halves. The top half of the character is "zhi" which means "to hold in one's hand, to keep, or to carry out." It alternatively represents a figure planting a tree or carefully working the soil. The radical for fire "huo" 火 is represented on the bottom by four short strokes, eloquently balancing the water element found in the "chao" character. The overall meaning of "re" is the "making or cultivation of fire." This is a beautiful explanation of the character, and cultivation is the key word here. It informs us of our innate ability to generate, cultivate, and control our internal environment… that is, ebb and flow, yin and yang.

"Re" 热 is a versatile and frequently used character in Chinese medicine. It's often used for describing heat symptoms, syndromes, disorders, disease, etc. When researching hot flashes, it is necessary to look towards not only the "re" 热 character to obtain a deeper understanding, but also the "huo" 火 character. The complexity and interchangeability of the two characters will become clear in the next chapters.

Huo 火: This is a literal pictograph of fire or flames. "Huo" can represent internal heat sources or pathogenic factors in Chinese medicine and its very essence is the culmination embedded in the characters for hot flash. After all, our understanding of fire within the body is the main objective of this book. To successfully treat hot flashes, we need to understand "huo." What is its source? Where does it originate? Why does it exist? What is its purpose? How can we control it? How can we utilize it? Why is it only apparent in certain women, at certain times, in certain locations? Why is it out of control in women only during menopausal transition? Why is it sometimes not easily controlled? Why does it ebb and flow on a daily or yearly cycle? We'll discuss and answer these questions in the chapters to come.

In conclusion, as we look at the definition of "chao re," we can begin to understand that it does accurately represent a hot-flash translation. But as we go deeper into the meaning of the two characters, we can see an interpretation describing the ebb and flow of yin and yang and the balance of water and fire that is the very essence of the hot flash and menopausal transition.

Heat and Fire—The Hot Flash

In the clinical setting, women of a wide range of ages and geographic, economic, educational, and societal backgrounds can present with hot flashes. These distinctly different individuals share one common trait—hot flashes. Based on Chinese medicine, we know hot flashes are the result of one or a multitude of simultaneous imbalanced internal mechanisms.

The hot flash is usually considered heat, hence the name. Heat is necessary for life. Heat warms, propels, and provides energy to every living cell. Our human body requires and relies on heat from both external and internal sources. Understanding our heat sources enables us to understand physiological heat versus pathologic heat.

It is easy to consider hot flashes as pathologic heat that needs to be extinguished. After all, they are not comfortable. In many cases though, hot flashes are a necessary symptom coming from internal and natural physiological processes. These types of processes are needed and required to bring yin and yang back into relative balance, to aid the formation of qi and blood, and to regulate the zangfu organs. Menopausal transition is often regarded as a sacred rebirth in women where the phoenix is rising from the ashes. Great energy is needed for this rebirth.

In our discussion, there may be confusion between the terms "heat" and "fire." In Chinese medicine, there are many nuances to both definitions, based on theory, pathology, and diagnostics. In some situations they may be synonymous, at other times they may be independent, and under various conditions they may be interchangeable or continuations. The main point to make clear here about the hot-flash environment is that the hot flash is a burst of qi rising to the surface, whether due to a natural physiological process or a pathologic situation. Whichever the case, the hot flash, as a symptom, is a feeling of heat or warmth. We will explore both the physiological and pathogenic natures generating this heat, and the similarities and differences between the terms heat and fire will become clearer.

We will consider normal heat sources within the body that are necessary for growth and survival. We will also discuss the natural balance of the body components and how their disruption and imbalance can create heat and fire. With this understanding, we can begin to look at the types of heat and fire and the many areas of the body in which they take place, including the zangfu organs. We'll also draw on many of the major classical Chinese-medicine books to see what they can contribute to our understanding of internal heat and fire as it relates to hot flashes. By taking a closer look at the body mechanics and how disequilibrium plays a part, we can better understand the components and build our understanding of the hot-flash environment to better help and treat the patient.

Sovereign Fire and Ministerial Fire

A proper heat source (yang) along with a proper nourishment source (yin) is a necessity for supporting life. Our body is no different and internally harbors both sources of yin and yang to support growth, development, and life. Two main internal heat sources are the sovereign fire and ministerial fire. The ministerial fire 相火 (xiang huo) is the fire that inhabits the life gate 命门 (mingmen), which resides in the lower abdomen between the kidneys. It stands in "complementary opposition" to the sovereign fire 君火 (jun huo), or the heart fire, which resides in the chest. As the ministerial fire moves upwards and outwards, the sovereign fire brings warmth inwards and downwards. Together, they mutually warm the zangfu organs and power the activity in the body.

The ministerial fire is the primary source of fire for the body, and when it is in balance, its yang energetic effects will warm the body and generate, propel, and supply the source (yuan) qi to the entire body. Ministerial fire can become overexuberant due to various lifestyle or internal factors affecting the zangfu organs, including an insufficiency of yin, an abundance of yang, damp-phlegm, and stagnation, creating an imbalance in the mingmen. It is thought that the ministerial fire can then become hyperactive and this fire in turn will flame upwards. The ministerial fire is also considered the fire of the pericardium developing from the lower jiao. Due to its intimate connection to the heart (yin) and pericardium (yang), a frenetic ministerial fire can gather in the heart and chest (the sovereign fire) to create one possible hot-flash environment scenario.

Pathogenic Heat and Fire

Heat, in general, can come from the exterior or the interior of the body. The external environment has the ability to invade the body. In general terms, we often think about viruses, bacteria, molds, etc. that cause colds, flu, seasonal allergies, and so on. I remember the warnings growing up... wear a jacket in the rain or you will catch cold... wear a hat so you don't lose heat in the cold weather... don't stay in the sun too long... stay hydrated... don't spend too much time in a damp environment or you'll catch pneumonia. These warnings stem from our understanding that the external environment has an effect on the internal health of the body. These, in Chinese medicine, are called the six excesses—wind, cold, summer-heat, damp, dryness, and fire—which invade from the exterior environment. The six excesses are also known as the six qi or six kinds of weather.

Fire and summer-heat are mere expressions of heat. Fire, heat, and warmth can also be viewed as mere expressions or intensities of each other. So when the weather is abnormally hot outside, or one is out for an abnormally long period of time in the hot weather, there is a potential for heat to invade the body and cause disease. Common symptoms include fever, sweating, thirst, desire for coolness, vexation, redness of the face, eyes, urine, or tongue, or a rapid pulse. Most healthy people can abate the symptoms in a short period of time by coming out of the heat and cooling down without long-standing symptoms or damage to the body. However, with long or repeated exposure, or when it happens to a body in weakened condition, the heat can invade the interior.

This brings the discussion to internal pathogenic heat. Internal pathogenic heat comes from the following issues: exposure to the external environment that allows heat to invade the body; the transformation of yang qi, as a result of a myriad of factors that can disrupt the qi dynamic, yinyang, and general physiological factors within the body. These factors of disruption may be due to intense or chronic emotional issues, dietary habits, physical and mental exhaustion, fatigue, and other lifestyle factors that strain one's internal physiological process and revitalization.

Once pathogenic heat invades or after it is internally generated inside the body, it will affect each tissue and organ system in a unique way, causing disruption, imbalance, weakness, or hyperactivity situations. In general, there are two types of pathogenic internal heat: repletion (excess) and vacuity (deficiency) heat/fire.

Deficiency and Excess

Deficiency or "vacuity" 虚 (xu) is "emptiness or weakness," while excess or "repletion" 实 (shi) is "fullness or strength" (Wiseman and Ye 1998, p.645). Repletion or excess patterns are the result of the natural resistance of the body to something abnormal either from the external or internal environment. It's the body's qi fighting off a pathogenic factor or its resistance to the natural physiology causing abnormally strong results or symptoms. Repletion heat or fire patterns are commonly due to exuberant evil heat affecting the digestive tract (yangming) and liver/gallbladder (shaoyang). These patterns are often the result of exposure to external pathogenic factors, irregular dietary habits (including contaminated food and water), or intense or strong emotional stimuli. Repletion fire/heat signs include high fever, aversion to heat, headaches, red eyes, bitter taste in the mouth, dry mouth, heart vexation, thirst, constipation, abdominal pain, yellow or concentrated urine, yellow tongue fur, and a forceful and rapid pulse.

Vacuity heat and fire patterns generally arise from the depletion of yin creating an exuberance of yang, or what I like to call "unchecked yang," that is an imbalance of yin and yang. The depletion of yin happens over a longer period of time from the natural aging process, chronic or severe illness, loss of blood, long-standing exposure to environmental or external pathogenic factors, long-standing mental-emotional issues, and other problematic lifestyle habits, where numerous qi dynamic imbalances slowly consume yin. These imbalances inevitably affect the zangfu organs, causing disruption to and further consumption of qi, blood, yin, yang, or essence. Once the vital qi has been damaged and the yin qi has been depleted, the yang qi will become unchecked, having the tendency to generate radiating low-grade heat symptoms. Vacuity heat signs include low-grade tidal fever, tidal redness in the face, vexing heat in the five palms, insomnia, reddish urine, dry mouth and throat, night sweating, a red tongue with no coating, and a fine and rapid pulse. It is largely thought that the terms "vexing heat" and "tidal fever" may apply to the same idea as the hot flash. Heart vexation, on the other hand, is thought of as a strong feeling of heat, unrest, irritability, or agitation in the heart region.

Vacuity Fire and Vacuity Heat

There is a subtle difference between vacuity fire and vacuity heat that must be addressed when we are diagnosing and treating hot flashes. Vacuity fire is a depletion of the true yin or kidney yin, while vacuity heat is a heat due to the insufficiency of yin humor (the makeup of the essence, blood, jin ye—liquid and humor) in contrast to unchecked yang qi. Essentially, one is a deficiency of an organ's ability to maintain normal levels of yin humor, while the other is the actual depletion of the body's yin source.

How to differentiate between the two is a common issue and can be problematic in the clinic since the former usually causes the latter. Primary kidney yin deficiency (vacuity fire) generally takes a longer aging time to fall deficient unless there are inherited genetic issues or a history of severe illness, trauma, or taxation. In terms of menopausal transition, based on my clinical experience, I don't believe this is necessarily the chief underlying cause of the hot flash. What I do see more often is general vacuity heat patterns generating the hot-flash symptoms, while the kidney yin may still be relatively intact. In fact, it may be likely there is an underlying kidney yang issue that is concurrent with general vacuity heat. This is because general yin deficiency can happen over a relatively shorter period of time and can affect any zangfu organ due to the myriad of lifestyle factors previously discussed.

This important understanding explains why when we're treating hot-flash patients, hot flashes will often be quelled more easily by nourishing the yin of the heart, stomach, or liver, in conjunction with fortifying the yin and yang of the kidney as a whole. One may even need to drain the kidney fire while simultaneously nourishing the yin of the other zangfu organs.

Heat and Fire Pathology

To conclude the discussion on heat and fire, let's focus on the formation and generation of internal heat and fire based on the disruption of the internal qi dynamic. The internal qi dynamic is the collection of physiological functions of all of the internal zangfu organs and the channel system. When the entire system is working in harmony and at its optimum, yin and yang will be harmonized, the yuan qi will be in abundance, and the qi and blood can flow freely without resistance. Natural life tendencies tend to interfere with our qi dynamic, creating deficiencies, excesses, and stagnations.

Qi dynamic interruptions are a natural part of the body, happen daily, and can be small or large based on the problem. For example, stagnation can merely be waiting for a red light or it may be due to a traffic jam. You're stopped for a portion of time and then able to move forward. The same thing happens within the body's physiological process. It is said that heat builds within the body from stagnation. Once the stagnation is gone, the heat is released. I sometimes think of it like a pressure cooker or a volcano releasing steam. Over time, these imbalances create many situations: the consumption of vital qi; the inability to generate new qi; yinyang imbalance; the generation of damp-phlegm, cold, and heat or fire. Many of the common individual scenarios will be discussed further in Chapter 2.

The hot-flash environment requires the practitioner to comprehend the physiological heat and fire within the body necessary to maintain health and the concepts behind the generation of pathogenic heat and fire. It is our job as Chinese-medicine practitioners to know these two concepts of physiological and pathogenic heat and fire and to understand where rebalancing and reestablishing of the two needs to happen in order to regain their balance for our patients' overall health.

Aspects of Qi

When we come to the realization that there are a multitude of energy currents within the body working simultaneously to support our existence, we as clinicians can begin to treat our patients. As previously stated, these currents are a combination of gravitational trajectories, ebbing and flowing tides, axis rotations, pendulums, bellows, electrical circuits, water evaporation and precipitation, and irrigation systems. Both Chinese medicine and Western science recognize and rely on these understandings, whether it's respiration, circulation, or physiological movement. Nothing is still—everything is in constant flux.

From the Chinese medical perspective, we'll investigate yinyang, essence, qi dynamic, blood, the zangfu organs, the channel system, and many others. A closer look at these concepts and how interrelated and interchangeable they are will allow us to better understand the hot-flash environment.

Pulses: Adapt, Interject, Influence, and Change

The universe has a pulse, a beat, a rhythm, a flow, as does the earth, sun, moon, and stars. Our body too has a genetic pulse, a life beat. Our breath, our heart, our mind, our spirit follow a natural and universal rhythm, individually and in unison with the environment as an orchestra. Our organs and tissues communicate with one another along with this beat… all in rhythm, ever-changing. Pulses, beats, frequency, tone—they all have yinyang. Yinyang pulsates and beats, changes, and is never constant.

There are certain beats we cannot control, as with universal beats. Yet there are others we have some control over, such as our breathing. Some take time to become aware of and to control, while others we control on a daily and consistent basis. All in all, many of these pulses we have the ability to "adapt" to, many we have the ability to "interject" with, and many we can "influence" and "change." Each individual has the unique opportunity to awaken to and experience this gift of life.

I believe there are several independent qi flows working in symbiosis within the body. An internal body qi flows to the beating rhythm of one's own body clock and the qi flow of the universe. The lung and kidney qi flows with a rhythmic breath. The heart and lung qi flows with smooth blood circulation. The liver and heart qi flows with a calm spirit. Every qi flow functions independently yet communicates with the others. None are in primary command, but they take cues from one another. Thinking of hot flashes as a "rebirth" or "second spring," perhaps they are the body's multiple qi flows adjusting and reestablishing to a new rhythm. Perhaps hot flashes are a minor inconvenience for some women because all of the qi flows balance quickly and easily without effort, while others suffer from severe or chronic hot flashes because there is one or multiple qi flows resisting balance or coming into rhythm.

The pulses do interplay and have an effect on each other. Not only can they have a positive effect, but they can also affect one another negatively.

We may find some qi pulses are weak while others are too strong. Interjecting with lifestyle modifications can help bring them into a more beneficial rhythm. The qi pulses within the body are susceptible to many influences throughout our lives and gradually lose strength, become too weak, fast, slow, or strong... and eventually they lose strength and cease.

Controlling the Tides

The ebb and flow of the qi in the body comes and goes like the tides. The qi, the blood, yin and yang rise and fall. They continuously move at the pace they are meant to, change over time, and are influenced by age and our personal lives. To understand the hot-flash environment requires understanding the changes in the tides in the body.

The Rise and Fall of Yin and Yang

Yin and yang is a qi mechanism within our body and designed for homeostasis. The yin and yang ebb and flow, rise and fall, daily within the body. One turns into the other, balancing one another's increase and decline in strength. Yang qi slowly begins to build just past midnight to reach its peak and maximum yang at midday. Midday then gives way for yin to build and grow where it eventually reaches its peak and maximum yin at midnight, when the cycle starts again. The two mutually support and balance their counterpart. The relative strength of the two changes throughout the day, through the aging process, and throughout our internal environment. Our internal zangfu organs are continuously supporting and balancing one another based on yin and yang theory.

The Balance of the Water and Fire

The internal ministerial fire rises from the mingmen in the lower abdomen to meet with the sovereign fire within the heart in the chest. The sovereign fire descends to meet with the ministerial fire within the mingmen. This rising and falling of fire is the balance of the lesser yin (shaoyin) and lesser yang (shaoyang). The ministerial fire is the rising yang (fire) within the yin (water) and the sovereign fire is the descending yin (water) within the yang (fire). The ministerial fire smolders within the mingmen and is employed to engender yin. The yin qi, with the help of the ministerial fire, rises to meet and is able to balance the sovereign fire and its forceful yang energy. The sovereign fire takes the external yang heat into the body and descends downwards to meet and support the ministerial fire. The two fires together mutually warm the zangfu organs and power the activity in the body.

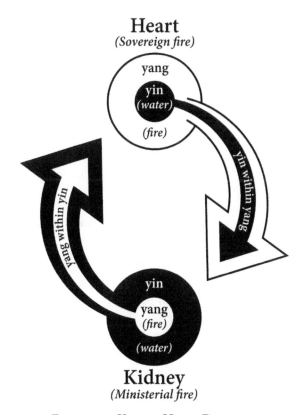

Heart
(Sovereign fire)

yang
yin
(water)

(fire)

yin within yang

yang within yin

yin
yang
(fire)

(water)

Kidney
(Ministerial fire)

FIGURE 1.2: KIDNEY-HEART DYNAMICS

Dual Shaoyin

The two shaoyin organs within the body are the heart and the kidney. The heart resides within the chest and the kidney resides in the lower abdomen. It is said that their relationship is a balance of water and fire. The kidney belongs to the water phase and the heart belongs to the fire phase. The kidney water rises to cool the heart fire and the heart fire descends to warm the kidney water. Together, they bring yinyang balance to the yin humor, zangfu organs, sensory organs, and tissues throughout the body.

Yin Within Yang—Yang Within Yin

It is said that when either yin or yang reaches its absolute that it turns into the other. The lower jiao (mingmen) is yin to the upper jiao (chest) that is yang. Yang rises, yin falls. Yang rises to help spread yin throughout and to nourish the body. Then, it descends back to the original source to engender more yin. The yang travels up within the yin and descends with the help of yin within yang. The yin cannot rise without the forceful power of yang. The yang cannot descend without the heavy downward flow of the yin. If one is too weak or too strong, the balance is upset.

Water Over Fire

Found within the *Yi Jing* 易经 (*The Book of Changes*), Hexagram 63, "jì jì" 既濟 illustrates water over fire (yin over yang): "Water's [yin] nature is downward flowing, and fire's [yang] nature is upward burning" (Wang 2012, p.69). This is the opposite of the water and fire balance of the kidney and heart. Water and fire, like yin and yang, merge together and transform to promote each other. This is mutual harmonization and assistance and beautifully demonstrates the sustained balance of thermoregulation in the body.

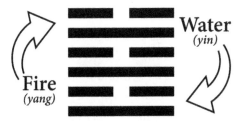

FIGURE 1.3: JÌ JÌ DYNAMICS

The Breathwork of the Greater and Lesser Yin

Inhalation is yin and exhalation is yang. Our breath works like a great bellows, continually generating and moving qi and blood throughout the body. Upon inhalation, the lung (taiyin) gathers the air (da qi) within it and in turn the kidney (shaoyin) grasps hold of it and leads the qi downwards to receive it. Within the kidney, the air qi combines with the essential (jing) qi. Upon exhalation, the movement is reversed. The kidney releases the newly engendered qi upwards to combine with the food and drink (gu qi) within the spleen (taiyin) to create the source (yuan) qi, which arrives back in the chest where it becomes the true (zhen) qi. This principle is what I call the "axis of life" or the lung-spleen-kidney axis. This axis is of utmost importance, for the inhalation and exhalation of the breath generates and circulates qi and blood.

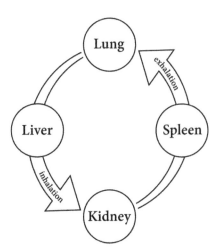

FIGURE 1.4: LUNG AND KIDNEY—BREATH DYNAMICS

The Chong Mai

The chong mai (penetrating vessel) is known as the sea of blood. It is the deepest vessel in the body and the center for the entire channel system. It supplies the uterus with blood and controls menstruation. It is at the heart of menopausal transition.

The chong mai originates in the uterus and its three branches span upwards through the three jiao to the chest and face, through the spine, and downwards along the leg to the sole of the foot. Its yang motive forces rise up along the stomach, kidney, and shaoyang channels. Its yin nutritive forces descend along the kidney, spleen, and liver channels.

The chong mai balances a confluence of interior with exterior, heart and kidney, and yin and yang. It is yin in nature yet yang in dynamic. It is susceptible to internal qi damage, fire, stagnation, and blood deficiency. The chong mai has a relationship with the san jiao, heart, and kidney fire, all linked to the ministerial fire. It is known as the great thoroughfare and has a surging property. If its qi cannot flow unimpeded, counterflow qi can ascend upwards along the stomach channel, kidney channel, or shaoyang channels to fill the chest, agitate the heart shen, and flare the heart fire, and present with abdominal urgency, agitation, and heat symptoms.

The sea of blood is abundant during a woman's reproductive years, but is slowly diminished over time by the continuous loss of blood from the monthly menstrual cycle. The chong mai is exhausted by the time a woman reaches menopausal transition. This cycle is in direct correlation with the ovarian reserve. A woman's body becomes increasingly blood (yin) deficient while a surplus of qi (yang) is abundant. The chong mai becomes less yin in nature and prone to yang influences with upsurging qi tendencies that can agitate the heart and shen. This foundational theory illustrates how blood deficiency is of primary importance in understanding hot flashes.

The Six Jing (Channels)

The six jing are the rising and falling of yin and yang. Their continual circular motion maintains homeostasis within the body. When one or more of the six jing become blocked or cannot maintain proper rhythm, disease results. Six-jing theory is discussed first in the *Huangdi Neijing Suwen* and is the backbone to the *Shang Han Lun*.

The three yang: Taiyang ascends upwards and outwards. Yangming descends downwards and inwards. These two represent the dueling rising and falling physiological yang activities within the body. Shaoyang, the third yang, functions to bring yang qi into the mingmen. This supports ministerial fire to "pivot" or generate and transform into yin qi.

The three yin: The three yin work primarily to bring warmth, yin, blood, and nutrition upwards to the zangfu organs and tissues of the body. Taiyin absorbs yang qi and generates yin. Shaoyin receives, absorbs, and stores yin. Jueyin is the upward movement of yin.

Nutrition and Defense
The wei (defensive) qi and the ying (nutritive) qi are the yin and yang of the true (zhen) qi. The wei qi is yang and the ying qi is yin. The wei qi flows upwards and outwards to protect the body, while the ying qi flows within the vessels to bring nourishment to the body. It is said that during the daytime, the wei qi rises to the surface, and during the nighttime, it descends back to the internal realm. This is the natural ebb and flow of yin and yang.

These descriptive concepts of yin and yang, water and fire, and qi and blood can help us better understand the aspects of qi within the body. The hot-flash environment can materialize from an imbalance of any one of these mechanisms. And even though all of these mechanisms work in harmony and mirror one another in function, it can happen that only one will fall out of balance while the others seemingly remain in perfect working order. It is then necessary for the practitioner to decipher and be able to diagnose and treat the imbalance while the rest are maintained.

Aspects of Blood
Blood is a major component in overall body health and it is very important for acupuncturists and Chinese-medicine practitioners

to understand its role in the hot-flash environment. I remember, early in my studies, my professor, Dr. Hong Chen, a third-generation Chinese-medicine dermatologist, saying that treating skin disorders effectively always comes back to treating the blood. Another Chinese-medicine mentor mirrored this thought in a lecture emphasizing the importance of supporting healthy blood for treating women's health issues. On both occasions, these concepts struck a resonance within my curiosity and I've carried them into my clinical practice, focusing my efforts on blood health, production, and movement. At its roots, Chinese medicine comes back to the basics of qi and blood.

Blood Formation

The pre-heaven qi stored in the kidney combines with the post-heaven qi generated primarily by the spleen and lung to make up the yuan (source) qi, the work of the axis of life or the lung-spleen-kidney axis. The yuan qi, the most basic form of qi in the body, consists of both yin and yang and is the primary source for what we call qi and blood. Qi and blood are yin and yang counterparts. Blood is a product of qi and is the warmth and nutrition for all tissues in the body. It is paramount to balance work and rest and to have good diet and exercise habits to maintain optimal production of the lung-spleen-kidney axis, while the partnership of the lung and heart organs help spread both qi and blood throughout the body. With the help of the liver-spleen-heart triad, there will be proper storage, production, and circulation of blood. When the blood is abundant and flourishing, the spirit is calm and emotions are stable.

It is necessary for us to understand and take this information to heart, for it explains so much and clears up unnecessary confusion when considering the many components of the hot-flash environment. First, all qi (and blood) within the body stems from the yuan qi. This is refreshing for me because when I'm working with patients, I know that whatever and wherever the problem is within the body, it is all interconnected by qi that comes from the same source. Second, the source qi comes from the three organs that generate qi: the lung-spleen-kidney axis. The continuous need to generate qi and supplement these three main organs never ceases in practice.

Spirit and Blood

It is said that the spirit resides in the blood. It is also said that the spirit resides in the heart and that the heart is the emperor of the body and ruler of the blood:

> The blood resides in the vessels; it is tied to the heart. Su wen 26 states: "Blood and qi are man's spirit. The spirit, though, is the ruler of the heart." From this it is evident that all the blood is tied to the heart. (Unschuld and Tessenow 2011, p.190)

The heart plays a major role in the hot-flash environment, which means there is a direct connection among hot flashes, the spirit, and the blood. To treat hot flashes, the blood needs to be addressed. A primary focus is to nourish the blood so it can calm and protect the spirit and nourish the heart. We treat the blood by nourishing and regulating the kidney-liver-spleen triad. Once imbalances in these organs are addressed and regulated, they can generate and build strong blood that will in turn balance the yin and yang within the heart, quelling the hot flashes.

Blood—Yin and Yang Components

Taking a closer look at blood, we can break it down into yin and yang components. The blood itself is yin by nature and, as we have already mentioned, serves as the nutrition for the tissues and organs. It also warms the tissues and organs, which serves as a yang function. If we dig even deeper into the blood, it is yin in nature because we can see and touch it, but also yang in nature, based on its invisible energetic and physiological nature. Employing the ying qi and wei qi theory, the ying qi nourishes the body (yin), while the wei qi warms and protects the body (yang).

The wei qi, however, is more relevant in the timing and times of day hot flashes are experienced. The wei qi is not necessarily considered the yang propellant of the yin or ying qi. Therefore, what exactly propels the yin? The yang warming function and propulsion of blood comes from inside, meaning the yang is within the yin. The yang fire within the yin water (blood) is another key component in explaining the hot-flash environment.

The natures of yin and yang are balanced relatively equally, even though they ebb and flow into each other throughout the course of a day. By superimposing this model onto the blood, the yang within the yin generally should be equal in strength and quantity. Over time, whether its genetics (congenital issues), chronic disease, lifestyle habits, aging, or in particular the menstrual cycle, the yin and yang qi of the blood will naturally fall out of balance, leaving either the yin or yang weaker or stronger. To utilize this theory to explain the source of hot flashes, there are two probable scenarios that will create a hot-flash environment—yin deficiency or yang exuberance.

The Yin and Yang Dynamic Within the Blood

I like to think of the yang within yin blood model much like I do an electrical cord. The copper wire contained inside the cord carries the electricity (yang) and the rubber casing encapsulates and protects the wire (yin). The two models can demonstrate how the yin and yang dynamic inside the blood can create a hot flash. Either the yin is weak, meaning that the rubber casing has worn thin, exposing the wire, or the yang is too strong, meaning the wire is drawing too much current; either of the two cases can generate heat, and both scenarios can explain a hazardous potential.

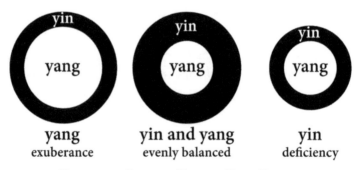

FIGURE 1.5: BLOOD—YIN AND YANG DYNAMICS

This theory is represented in Figure 1.5, and we can see a balanced yin and yang within the blood in the center model. It is clear that the yang (fire) within the blood is contained within the yin (water). However, if yang becomes exuberant or if yin becomes deficient, the threshold between the internal yang and the blood exterior becomes thin. The narrowing of the yin aspect of blood is similar to the narrowing of the body's thermoneutral zone regulated by the hypothalamus. The closer yang qi is to the surface of the blood, the easier it is for yang to intensify heat in the body.

Therefore, balancing the blood and quelling the hot flash requires cooling of the blood by nourishing or enhancing the yin, meaning enhancing the insulation of the power cord, and by reducing the yang, meaning drawing less power through the cord.

In the traditional sense, hot flashes have long been thought of as a result of a yin deficiency. But what type, and where is this deficiency? It has commonly been attributed to the kidney and perhaps the liver yin. The kidney not only act as the body's source of yin and yang, but also in modern times and Western thought are in relation to the ovaries. When the ovaries and estrogen are in decline, it is easy to think that the hot flashes are a result of kidney yin diminishment.

In my experience, though, there are several zang-organ yin deficiency scenarios that could also create a hot-flash environment and I don't necessarily buy into the concept that every menopausal woman suffers kidney yin deficiency.

Second, yang excess has also been thought of as a source of hot flashes, and often in conjunction with yin deficiency, which creates a similar scenario. Blood, on the other hand, is systemic, can be equally damaged in every woman in our society, and is another possible scenario. These scenarios explain several things: why some hot flashes fail to respond to yin nourishing herbal formulas but do respond to blood tonics; why women experiencing hot flashes, in conjunction with poor dietary habits and digestion, tend to have qi and blood deficiency symptoms; why many women with hot flashes don't present with yin deficient signs.

Consider a different scenario. What if the yin is relatively intact while the yang inside the blood is in excess? This creates a situation where the blood is heated by yang exuberance within. This exuberance is often more congenital, meaning these patients naturally have it, but becomes noticeable during menopausal transition when the blood yin declines just the right amount, exposing the heat. This scenario explains why many hot-flash patients will respond better to yang sedating and fire cooling formulas. These patients have the potential to suffer from long-term hot flashes.

Treating deficient yin is often correct, as long as you see blood as part of yin. One may argue that there are many herbs that tonify both yin and blood within the yin tonifying tonics and that you can treat them both at the same time. From my experience, however, I have found that some hot flashes respond better to herbal formulas primarily focused on nourishing and cooling the blood, leaving me to speculate that perhaps the kidney-tonifying herbs are unnecessary. I feel that sometimes it takes a longer aging process, a situation of congenital yin deficiency, or a chronic illness to severely deplete yin, but on the other hand, blood is easily depleted by the monthly menstrual cycle and lifestyle habits.

Blood Quality

Blood quality comes from a good diet, hydration, a lack of pharmaceuticals and chemicals, and proper circulation from some regimen of activity and meditation. I normally suggest walking and yoga for patients who don't have a physical lifestyle. These benefit the lung-spleen-kidney axis and the generation of qi and blood and also benefit the heart and calm the spirit. Patients with poor diets, including processed foods, sugars, dairy, salts, preservatives, and even over-supplementation, can develop unhealthy and sluggish blood. This type of blood has the potential to cause many problematic and systemic issues. Changing these negative inputs is paramount.

My point is, the blood nourishes every single cell of the body and supplies the brain. If the blood is of poor quality, the currents within the entire body, over time, will not function optimally. The metaphor of needing to change the oil in your car comes to mind—if you don't, the oil gets thick, dirty, and old, and the engine wears out more quickly, overheats, and eventually breaks down. Many times, the

Chinese medical practitioner (and the patient) will think the problem is a zangfu organ issue, but I'm convinced that it's really a lifestyle issue and is no fault of the heart, liver, kidney, lung, or spleen. A history of poor lifestyle habits will inevitably damage a woman's blood, thus creating an internal environment that is much more difficult to treat, especially during menopausal transition.

The hormones too are distributed via the bloodstream, and the brain is nourished by blood. From the Western medical point of view, hot flashes are due to the diminished ovarian reserve leading to a drop in estrogen, which in turn causes dysregulation within the hypothalamus, disrupting its ability to control body thermoregulation. When the blood is healthy and flows well through the vessels, it is much easier to regulate and quell hot flashes.

Over time, some women will naturally become blood deficient by the time they reach menopause simply because they either started life deficient (genetic or congenital), consumed or damaged blood over time (illness or menstrual history), or were unable to rebuild strong blood (diet and lifestyle habits). Treating hot flashes requires nourishing the blood quality and quantity, and balancing the yin and yang within the blood.

The key takeaway here is understanding that the quality, quantity, and overall health of the blood may be the key to why some women experience hot flashes during menopausal transition while other women do not.

Aspects of Yin and Yang

In Chinese medicine, we utilize the concept of yin and yang in many ways to understand health. Two concepts are primary. First, yin and yang as components of the qi, the main physiological component for the zangfu organs and tissues, and second, yin and yang as a diagnostic tool to describe the function of the zangfu organs, qi and blood, essence, senses, spirit, and so on. If these two yin and yang concepts are not understood and delineated, confusion will arise in the clinical setting with understanding pathology, developing a correct diagnosis and treatment strategy, and administering the proper treatment.

For example: A patient is suffering from hot flashes and fatigue. Since the hot flashes make her feel hot all of the time, the practitioner diagnoses her with some form of heat or excess yang qi and prescribes heat clearing and yang sedating herbs or acupuncture treatments. But what if the patient does not feel any sustained relief? I believe in the power of acupuncture and the healing capability of the body, so when patients receive acupuncture, the body will naturally start (or at least try) to move in a positive health trajectory. But if the treatment strategy and treatments are not correct, the patient will only receive temporary relief and will inevitably slip back into the old trajectory.

In this hypothetical case, the true diagnosis is qi and yang deficiency that is unable to generate and move new qi and blood. Without the new generation of qi and blood, the patient feels fatigue. When qi and blood don't move, they stagnate and then transform into heat, thus the hot flashes along with fatigue. One could argue that the excess heat is consuming the qi and blood, so by clearing heat, the qi and blood will be able to regenerate. If this is the case, the herbal and acupuncture treatments would be effective and the patient would experience improvement. The proper treatment would then be to tonify qi and yang, while appropriately quelling the fire. With this treatment, the patient feels more energy and her hot flashes subside. This is, in fact, a common hot-flash patient presentation in the clinic. This demonstrates how vital it is to understand the concepts of yin and yang and how to use these concepts effectively to improve clinical success.

The majority of common and natural hot flashes, in my clinical opinion, are the result of unchecked yang rising upwards and dispersing outwards in the form of heat. The heat is not always or necessarily a pathogenic heat but merely bursts of qi manifesting as heat internally generated from the hot-flash environment. The theory behind the effulgent yang is a disruption to the balance in the natural ebb and flow of the internal yin and yang cycle. Hot flashes are triggered by a myriad of disruptions (excesses and deficiencies) within the body, and the pathology behind these disruptions is the diagnostic question we are seeking to answer.

There is a finer and more delicate balance of the yin and yang by the time menopausal transition arrives. Yin, which is intimately connected to blood, has gone through substantial and ongoing challenges throughout a woman's life, mainly due to the constant need for regeneration from the monthly menstrual cycle. It is natural for yin and blood to become deficient. The yang too must work overtime to help support the regeneration of this yin and blood, and it too can become exhausted. This explains the importance of a woman maintaining and supporting the yin and yang over the decades of monthly menstrual cycles. Proper diet, exercise, rest, stress management, joy, and purpose in life all help maintain and generate yin and yang qi. It is easy to understand that this can be very challenging and the multiple challenges women face in modern society are probably why hot flashes and other menopausal transition symptoms are more problematic nowadays.

Both the pre-heaven qi and post-heaven qi will have affected the balance of yin and yang in every woman by the time she has reached menopausal transition. It is up to the practitioner to understand the unique development of this process in each patient's lifespan to understand their hot-flash environment.

Scenarios of Yin and Yang Imbalance

The yinyang symbol "taijitu" denotes the balance of yin and yang, with the yin (black) sinking downwards and the yang (white) rising upwards. Yin and yang are in constant motion throughout nature and within our body. One rises and the other falls; one reaches its zenith and then transforms into the other; each generates the other; each nourishes the other; each controls the other; each is rooted in the other. This is the way of qi within the body and the universe.

Rise and Descent

There are two dueling processes of yin and yang: the rise of yin and the descent of yang, and the rise of yang and the descent of yin. This can be confusing in the discussion of hot flashes because the two are in opposition. But with closer analysis, it becomes clear. The former explains the physiological need of the kidney water (yin) to ascend to balance the heart fire (yang), which in turn descends to warm the kidney water (yin). The latter explains the physiological need of the kidney fire (yang) to ascend along with the kidney water (yin), helping it warm and spread the nutritive qi throughout the body; while the heart water (yin) descends along with the heart fire (yang), helping it cool and regulate the mingmen (this is illustrated in Figure 1.2).

When treating the hot-flash environment, it is necessary to understand that both yin and yang flow simultaneously together, so in effect there are two sets, a pair of yin and yang ascending and, at the same time, a pair of yin and yang descending. Effective treatment of problematic hot flashes focuses on the imbalance of excess and deficiency within the rising and falling pairs.

Yang Deficiency

The first concept in understanding yang deficiency starts within the mingmen in the lower abdomen where the generation of yin (water) takes place. The yang (fire) needs to descend and bring warmth from the environment down to the mingmen to generate yin. Without yang, yin cannot be born. Newly generated yin is vital and needs to rise up from the mingmen to nourish the zangfu organs and spread to all tissues throughout the body.

The yang qi is necessary to generate yin, much like a fire is needed beneath water to bring it to a boil. New yin cannot be generated, nor can it rise, without the ascending potential and the natural propulsion of yang. If the yang qi is weak, there will not be enough fire to accomplish this goal, leading to slower yin generation. This scenario, over time, leads to sluggishness and stagnation, with the eventual generation of heat or fire (yin fire) within the mingmen that can result in creating a hot-flash environment.

Clearly, the cause of this type of hot flash is yang deficiency. The question then becomes whether this is because yang qi failed to descend or because there is a true yang deficiency in the mingmen. The main focus for diagnosing this scenario is on the overall strength of yang qi in the upper body (sovereign) and lower body (mingmen). Diagnosing the cause of hot flashes requires looking beyond the heat signs. A patient with an exuberance of yang qi above that is failing to descend will present with many accompanying excessive yang symptoms and the exuberance will be apparent in the tongue and pulse, while a yang deficiency below will present as quite the opposite, with other general yang, qi, and blood deficiency symptoms.

Yang Excess

Now let's consider the reverse pathology, an excess of yang qi. Exuberant yang qi within the mingmen is like a high and intense flame rapidly boiling water resulting in the consumption of water and steam. In this situation yin is not properly generated, but consumed by the excessive yang fire. The result is less yin (water) and more yang (steam). Yang without the anchoring effect and adequate supply of yin will rise at a faster pace. The consequence is the rapid rising and propulsion of yang with a less than adequate yin supply. This not only results in the yin malnourishment of the organs and tissues, but also, the exuberant yang harassing the organs and upper portions of the body. This is another hot-flash environment scenario. The diagnostic distinction to make in this situation is whether there was an exuberance of yang within the mingmen to start with, or was there an overabundance of yang qi descending into the mingmen?

Imbalance of yin and yang, under normal circumstance, does not develop overnight, but over longer periods of time. In the case of yang excess in the mingmen, this type of patient would have had apparent yang excess symptoms prior to perimenopause and menopausal transition. The same is true for the case of excess yang in the upper regions.

But there are other scenarios that can more abruptly create yang excess above or below. A patient with an acute yang excess situation would likely have experienced something recently, such as having been exposed to hotter than normal temperatures or environments, having been through acute or severe emotional issues, or having digested alcohol, or rich and spicy, hot, unsanitary, or other improper foods, that quickly allowed yang qi to accumulate in the sovereign or mingmen. These possibilities are not pathologically systemic and should respond quite well to treatment.

Both scenarios can generate hot flashes. The former is seen in the type of patient that has suffered from long-standing heat issues, while the latter stems from more acute and sudden heat issues. With careful inquiry into the patient's history, the practitioner will be able to delineate between the two.

Yin Deficiency

Yin qi deficiency is the hallmark pathomechanism in the hot-flash environment. In most cases of problematic hot flashes, there is a yin deficient component. This occurs because of a sequence of natural events. Throughout the part of a woman's life leading up to menopausal transition, the yin and yang dichotomy slowly changes and naturally falls out of balance. In Chinese medicine, it is said that the essence (jing) of the body declines with age. Within the essence is yin qi and yang qi, therefore there too is a natural decline of the yin and yang. It's uncertain, though, whether one will decline more than the other. This is usually based on the predisposition of the woman's pre-heaven qi and partly on her lifestyle traits, her post-heaven qi.

Yin and blood are of the same source, and throughout the decades of monthly menstrual cycles there is a constant need for regeneration. This results in a natural potential for yin and blood to become deficient. With an environment of yin deficiency, a process of imbalance develops. First, the deficient yin is unable to anchor yang, which allows the natural tendency of yang to more easily rise and float upwards from the mingmen. Conversely, without enough yin in the sovereign to lead the yang qi downwards, yang will naturally remain in the upper regions of the body. Finally, without the sufficient nourishment and cooling functions of the yin, zangfu organs and tissues throughout the body become malnourished and overheated. The resulting pattern is a consistent ascending flow of yang qi, along with the deficiency of yin (water) unable to quell the yang (fire), leading to the unopposed creation of heat that resides in the sovereign, thus creating the typical hot-flash environment. It is very common to see simultaneous yin deficiency and yang excess patterns.

Yin Excess

Our final scenario is yin excess. Although not as common as other scenarios, yin excess has the potential to create the hot-flash environment. Yin excess has the tendency to descend and suppress or consume yang qi. One hot-flash scenario happens when excess yin subdues yang qi. This increases the difficulty of the yin and yang to maintain the smooth flow of qi, blood, and body fluids and can lead to their stagnation and accumulation. Stagnation and accumulation have the potential to generate heat or fire, and, over time, create a hot-flash environment. Another hot-flash possibility occurs where yin excess accumulates within the mingmen due to yang deficiency. This excess yin will upsurge. The true yang stored within the mingmen will rise along with the excess yin. The true yang eventually will reach and harass the heart fire. This concept is discussed in greater detail in Chapter 3. It is more common to see yin excess in conjunction with yang deficiency.

Applying Yin and Yang Balance to Diagnosis and Treatment

The theory of yin and yang balance is at the core of understanding the hot-flash environment. Detriment to yin affects yang. Detriment to yang affects yin. A deficit of one naturally leads to a surfeit of the other, while a surfeit of one will weaken the other. It is typical to see combinations of excess and deficiency yin and yang situations in the clinical setting. Any and all of the imbalances of yin and yang can result in setting up the hot-flash environment.

Traditional hot-flash treatment based solely on draining fire and clearing heat will often be ineffective and may even be detrimental to the patient's health. An approach based on yin and yang will include enriching yin, subduing or fostering yang, and generating a proper flow of qi and blood to quell or subdue fire. My research and clinical experiences show that this approach is significantly more effective.

Wei Qi

What role does the wei qi 卫气 "defensive qi" or "guard qi" play in hot-flash physiology? The defensive qi carries the generalized function of protecting the body from the environment and external pathogens, including changes in the weather, viruses and other things that cause illness, and other environmental issues that can cause harm to our body. But it also has the ability to warm, moisten, and nourish the skin and muscles, and control the opening and closing of skin pores. This is in contrast to the functions of the ying qi 营气 "nutritive qi," "construction qi," or "camp qi," which travels within the blood vessels, along with the blood, to nourish and replenish the body tissues and zangfu organs. These theories are accentuated in the *Neijing Lingshu* where it states:

> Those floating qi that do not move along the conduits, they are the guard qi. The essence qi that move in the conduits, they are the camp qi. (Unschuld 2016a, p.501)

The wei qi is yang and floats in the surface between the skin and muscles. From this body region, yang qi warms, controls, and protects the surface of the body from the exterior environment. While I do not believe wei qi is directly responsible for causing hot flashes, I do believe it plays a role in the hot-flash environment. It may be disrupted or disrupting to the body due to a long course of disharmonies in the body, thus leading to the hot flashes and sweating issues in menopausal-transition patients. Since wei qi is yang in nature and has an intimate relationship with controlling body temperature and sweating, it is certainly worth investigation.

Wei Qi Dysfunction

What causes a disruption in the wei qi? First, consider the origin and function of the defensive qi. The defensive qi is a piece of the qi system. It is derived from the combination of the essential (jing) qi of the kidney and the food (gu) qi from the spleen. In the chest, it's refined into the true (zhen) qi. The zhen qi spreads throughout the entire body and can be broken into its yin component ying (nutritive) qi and yang component wei (defensive) qi.

The yang nature of wei qi is naturally balanced by the yin nature of ying qi. The strength and flow of wei qi is influenced by yinyang excess and deficiencies and the existence of heat or fire.

Like any qi, excess heat or yang exuberance will drastically increase propulsion of qi, making it frantic, irregular, and uncontrollable. We can theorize that this is the result of internal issues of heat or hyperactive yang due to excess or deficiency situations. Excess conditions result in bigger results and can conceivably be the source of constant hot flashes throughout the day or hot flashes lasting many years beyond menopausal transition. This may affect not only the frequency, but also the duration and severity.

Deficiency issues often play a leading role with qi. Without the foundation of yin, blood, and jing, the qi has nothing to anchor to and naturally floats about. The wei qi will wander to and fro without the leadership of the yin substance. The wei qi will rise to the surface at times when yin qi is especially weak in the afternoon and evening. The wei qi can be controlled once the therapy is directed towards nourishing the blood, yin, and jing. Deficiency and excess conditions are commonly seen in hot-flash patients and can increase or escalate severity and chronicity.

In contrast, sometimes it is the yang qi components of the zangfu organs that are weak and unable to generate enough ying qi. The manifestations of heat are the result of deficient ying qi (yin) allowing an abundance of wei qi (yang). The more deficient the ying qi becomes, the more pulsation of the wei qi is felt within the body as heat.

Stagnations too can disrupt the natural flow of qi. Stagnations from the zangfu organs, particularly the liver and the digestive tract, will generate heat like a pressure cooker, releasing bursts of qi or heat as it builds and releases pressure. The clinical results are earlier hot flashes during perimenopause, or intense and long-standing hot flashes, frequent abating and reoccurring hot flashes, and irregular-patterned hot flashes.

Ying qi (yin) and wei qi (yang) are two parts of the zhen qi and the product of both pre-heaven and post-heaven qi. Supporting the zhen qi means supporting the lung-spleen-kidney axis and should be the first focus when treating hot flashes. By treating these three organs, we remediate the deficiency with nourishment. By regulating the yin and yang of the body, we can control the daily wei qi cycle. By treating stagnations, we allow the wei qi to flow freely.

In the past, I believed we could diagnose hot flashes purely on the ebb and flow of wei qi throughout the course of the day and treat them by sedating the yang qi. Based on my clinical experience, I have come to the conclusion that hot flashes are more related to the overall abundance and strength of the ying qi and its ability to contain the wei qi.

Chapter 2

Hot Flashes—Zangfu Organ Theory

Zangfu Organ Associations

The hot flash is a burst of qi, with the end result being the manifestation and feeling of heat rushing upwards and outwards to the surface of the body. Presumably, the understanding and effective treatment of hot flashes should be centered on heat/fire and its source. The feeling of heat is merely the manifestation. In order to treat the hot-flash environment, we need to understand the source of it.

The hot-flash environment comes into being from many factors developing over time and the way they simultaneously align during menopausal transition. Congenital factors, yin and yang, qi and blood, zangfu organs, and lifestyle habits will align just so in certain women.

Acupuncturists and Chinese-medicine practitioners have come to understand that the zangfu organs and their five phases are a primary source of dysfunction in the body. Discussing the zangfu organs, their relationships, and imbalances can shed some light on the source and creation of the hot-flash environment.

The Organs

Most modern Chinese medical texts and clinical manuals primarily base the theory of menopausal transition and hot flashes on the classic passage of the *Neijing* discussed earlier regarding women aging in seven-year increments until the age of 49. It is understood that when women are youthful, their kidney essence is strong and supportive, the tiangui or menstrual yin is full, the ren and chong vessels are open and flourishing, and the liver is full of blood. As women reach menopausal transition, the kidney essence is depleted, tiangui is exhausted, the ren and chong vessels are empty and no longer flow, and the liver is no longer filled with blood. The natural functions of menstruation and fertility slowly decline and cease. This is the natural physiological change in women.

The central zangfu organ during menopausal transition, and throughout a woman's life for that matter, is the kidney because of its ability to communicate and generate qi and blood along with the other zangfu organs.

The Kidney—The Foundation

The kidney is situated within the lower abdomen, form the mingmen, and are the foundation for the rest of the zangfu organs. They have an intimate connection to the ministerial fire, uterus, ovaries, and reproduction in both women and men, as well as a special relationship with the brain. The kidney, besides having a wide variety of functions, is the primary organ to support the true yin and yang and stores the essence (jing).

The kidney's true yin is the root of all yin in the body. Kidney yin supports, moistens, and nourishes the zangfu organs, sensory organs, and tissues throughout the entire body. Kidney yin deficiency will affect other organs (and vice versa), particularly the liver, heart, and lung, and will give rise to hyperactive yang, fire, and wind. Common yin deficiency signs during menopausal transition include tidal heat effusion, night sweating, insomnia with vivid dreams, excessive libido, dizziness, anxiety, generalized dryness symptoms, a red tongue, and a fine and rapid pulse.

The kidney's true yang is the root of all yang in the body. Kidney yang warms and activates the zangfu organs and the rest of the body. Insufficiency of kidney yang will disturb the water metabolism, re-productive function, and other organ functions, especially the spleen, heart, and lung. Common yang deficiency signs during menopausal transition include an aversion to cold, cold hands and feet, fatigue, body aches and pain, a pale tongue, and a weak pulse.

The kidney essence is the root and foundation of both yin and yang within the body. Yin and yang are interdependent and mutually counterbalancing. One affects the other. Imbalance of yin and yang is fundamentally attributed to essence deficiency.

During youth, the kidney is strong and essence is abundant. With age, the kidney essence naturally declines. The kidney essence is slowly consumed over time and becomes increasingly deficient. During menopausal transition, along with the natural decline of the kidney essence, the yin and yang of the kidney can also naturally decline and fall into disharmony. The decline of the kidney essence and yin and yang will create imbalances of the zangfu organs. Excess and deficiency patterns of qi, blood, yin, yang, fire, spirit, damp-phlegm, stagnation, and stasis arise.

The classic and primary kidney deficiency herbal formula is Liu Wei Di Huang Wan 六味地黄丸 (Six Ingredient Rehmannia Pill). Its actions are to enrich yin and nourish the kidney. The textbook kidney deficiency acupuncture formula is: BL23 (Shenshu) 肾俞, RN4 (Guanyuan) 关元, KI3 (Taixi) 太溪, BL52 (Zhishi) 志室, KI6 (Zhaohai) 照海, KI1 (Yongquan) 涌泉, SP6 (Sanyinjiao) 三阴交 (Wiseman and Ye 1998, p.336).

The Kidney and the Heart

The kidney (water) cannot balance thermoregulation on its own. It relies on the heart (fire) for balance, as we saw with Hexagram 63, "jì jì." The heart primarily functions to govern the blood and house the spirit. The heart is the sovereign of the zangfu organs and is positioned above them all in the chest.

The heart and kidney have a natural balance, connecting the upper and lower aspects. The kidney governs water and the heart governs fire. They are interdependent and counterbalance each other. The kidney water (yin) flows upwards to nourish the heart (yin) and quell the heart fire (yang). The heart fire (yang) descends to warm the kidney (yang) and generate kidney water (yin).

It can be natural for kidney yin to become deficient over time, especially in women, failing to support and quell the heart fire, which can then burn out of control and flare upwards. On the one hand, the kidney water becomes deficient and the fire within the heart blazes. On the other hand, if heart fire blazes from effulgence, the kidney water can be consumed, thus the balance is disrupted. This is called the non-interaction of the heart and kidney, a classical hot-flash scenario.

An imbalance between the kidney and heart can create deficiency or excess fire environments. Fire's natural tendency is to rise up, thus creating heat manifestations, pushing sweat from the body, and disturbing the heart spirit. The results are common menopausal-transition manifestations such as hot flashes, night sweats, sleep disorders (insomnia), heart palpitations, chest stuffiness, vexation, anxiety, and other emotional disorders.

The Heart—The Monarch

The heart is the sovereign of the zangfu organs and stores the spirit. The heart relies on qi, blood, yin, and yang nourishment from the rest of the zangfu organs, especially the kidney, spleen, and liver. The heart does not directly generate blood, even though it is the commander of blood. Deficiency of the source qi will ultimately affect the heart. However, when the heart qi and blood is full and abundant, it can function properly and the spirit will be clear and calm.

The heart has a special relationship to fire and this is of particular interest when talking about hot flashes. Based on five-phase theory, the heart belongs to fire. Positioned in the upper jiao it acts as a homing beacon for internal heat and fire. Once any internal bursts of qi, ascendant yang qi, or heat/fire find their way to the heart, via the zangfu organs, channel system, or directly from within the blood, they will agitate the heart fire. When the heart fire is set ablaze and exuberant, it will direct qi upwards and outwards towards the surface of the skin. This is the hot-flash mechanism. Theoretically, hot flashes are not directly heart fire—the heart is the conduit for the hot-flash release.

Though the heart is the monarch of the body, it is vulnerable to temporary and continuous harassment from both the external and internal environment. Various forms of environmental and emotional stimuli, and internal deficiency, excess, or stagnations, can have an impact on the heart fire and spirit and its ability to govern clearly.

The Kidney and the Liver

As with the heart, the kidney has a close and special relationship with the liver. The kidney stores essence and the liver stores blood. The kidney and the liver share the same origin. Essence and blood are both yin in nature. Blood is derived from the kidney essence and from the spleen qi. Together, the kidney and liver are mutually engendering and counterbalancing. A problem with one will inevitably affect the other. Insufficiency of the kidney essence or the liver blood will lead to dual liver and kidney yin deficiency.

Much like the kidney, the liver has its own natural balance of yin and yang contained within itself. The liver blood is yin while the liver qi is yang. The liver blood is on a continuous cycle of being stored during the nighttime and supplying the uterus and the rest of the body during the daytime. Conversely, the liver qi is constantly making sure that the zangfu organ and entire body's physiological process remains connected and in motion. There is no other place in the body where the balance of yin and yang is tested to this extreme on a daily basis.

There is a natural tendency, especially in women, for the liver yin or blood to become deficient, simply due to loss and regeneration from the monthly moon cycle. If that happens, there will be an imbalance of liver yin and yang, where the yang can become hyperactive and even generate fire. Liver yang hyperactivity or liver fire can then further damage the liver yin, blood, and kidney essence, creating a vicious cycle.

Liver (and kidney) yin deficiency will not be able to nourish the rest of the system, nor will it be able to subdue the yang. Hyperactive yang is ascending in nature and it will, with or without fire, harass the upper regions of the body. This disharmony can cause menopausal symptoms such as hot flashes, insomnia, and emotional upset, along with other common liver yang manifestations such as headaches, dizziness, and sensory organ disorders.

The Kidney and the Spleen and Stomach

Traditionally, we could stop the hot-flash environment explanation with the kidney-liver-heart trajectory. But in today's modern society and with the dietary habits of our industrialized nations, the kidney and spleen relationship must be addressed.

The spleen holds the center position of the zangfu organs and sits in the middle of the abdomen. The two chief organs in charge of digestion are the spleen and the stomach. They siphon the essence from the food and drink to generate qi and blood for the rest of the body, while the unusable portions are transformed into waste products. The activity of this process is yang in nature, while the end product is that of yin. These two organs are susceptible to excess and deficiency disorders. Deficiency patterns can lead to stagnation and repletion patterns and vice versa.

Yang is the fire and warming function of the body. The kidney yang is the spleen's main source of fire to transform food into qi and transport it to nourish the rest of the body. Without this warmth from the kidney yang, the spleen's functions will decrease and give rise to body fluid accumulation, qi stagnation, and blood stasis. This can create common menopausal-transition manifestations such as qi and blood deficiency symptoms including fatigue, insomnia, digestive problems, depression, and anxiety.

The spleen's central role of generating qi and blood and providing nourishment to the zangfu organs and the rest of the body is continual and paramount. The spleen and stomach are susceptible to worry, stress, overwork, and undernourishment, which slowly leads to spleen and stomach deficiency and the deficiency of qi and blood. This can be a slow process that may happen over years or decades. This weakened state depletes the liver blood and kidney essence and eventually causes a deficiency and imbalance of yin and yang. This cycle, whether it happens rather quickly or over time, ultimately leads to the malnourishment of the heart, depriving the heart of qi and blood. This is a common hot-flash environment, and once in place, the system will begin to show signs of fatigue, digestive and emotional issues, and the development of heat signs, such as hot flashes and sweating issues.

The spleen and stomach are also susceptible to excess patterns.

Eating poor quality or improper foods, irregular eating habits, and generalized overeating can lead to food and qi stagnation within the stomach. These excess stagnant patterns, like a smoldering volcano, will generate heat or fire, and over time can damage the stomach yin. The stomach sits directly below the heart, only separated by the diaphragm. The nature of the stomach qi is to descend. When there is stagnation, heat, or fire within the stomach, the stomach qi will have the tendency to ascend and thus harass the heart and disturb the spirit. This is a common hot-flash pattern seen in the clinical setting.

If the stomach excess pattern persists, over time it will injure and weaken the spleen. A weakened spleen will further lose its control over the digestion and its ability to support the stomach, weakening the stomach and leaving it vulnerable to continued damage. Hence, consistent overeating or eating improper foods will lead to a weakened spleen.

The Kidney and the Lung

This is the final piece of the puzzle. The kidney and lung have a truly engendering relationship. These two organs are of the utmost importance for optimal zangfu organ function, as well as maintenance of proper qi and blood circulation throughout the body. Disconnect of the kidney and lung qi can lead to circulation issues of the qi, blood, and body fluids within the zangfu organ system and throughout the channel system, leading to stagnation issues and yin and yang disharmony. The underlying pattern is an individual or dual weakness of the kidney and lung qi.

When the lung cannot descend and loses its qi connection to the kidney, the liver takes control of rising yang qi. The lung becomes exuberant with qi, its dispersing actions flare, and sweating happens. Exuberant qi retained in the lung and upper jiao eventually sets the heart fire ablaze.

This type of hot-flash environment is quite common in today's society. The stimulation needed to connect the kidney qi and lung qi is either broken or blocked. This is simply due to the fact that, as a species, we are less inclined to have constant activity throughout the day to maintain the lung-kidney connection through proper respiration. Or, alternatively, the qi is blocked in the chest due to stagnation, which keeps the lung qi from descending to meet with the kidney qi because of the ever-increasing stress and anxiety society places upon us. For some women, merely increasing activity and respiration is the key, while for other women, meditation and proper breath work can help correct the situation.

The Kidney and the Lower Jiao

The kidney has a special relationship with and command over the lower jiao. The kidney resides in the lower jiao and is the commander of this area of the body below the navel. The kidney oversees both internal and external aspects, including the sexual organs, menstruation, uterus, bladder, and external genitalia. It is natural to have physiological disorders in the lower jiao once the kidney loses its control over this area. With dysfunction in the lower jiao, it is likely to see menopausal-transition symptoms such as urinary disorders, menstrual irregularities such as prolonged or heavy menses, irregular menses, and ceasing of menses, vaginal dryness, and sexual dysfunction or desire.

The Kidney and the Brain

The kidney stores and supplies essence to the brain (sea of marrow). This Chinese-medicine perspective makes the connection between the two. When the kidney essence is abundant and its vitality is strong, the sea of marrow will be filled and there will be clear thoughts and memory. It is an important concept that bridges Chinese and Western medicine, as this concept linking the kidney and brain roughly mirrors the HPO axis cycle.

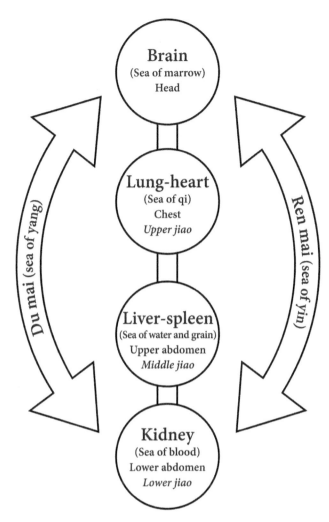

FIGURE 2.1: KIDNEY-BRAIN RELATIONSHIP

Conclusion

The zangfu system is a complex system to address since each mechanism affects and is affected by another component. When understanding, diagnosing, and treating the hot-flash environment, the initial step is to address the immediate symptoms by clearing heat, removing stagnation, and engendering the deficiency. This is only a short-term solution for many women.

Additional lifestyle changes and continued treatments addressing the necessary patterns are warranted. Positive lifestyle changes pose a low health risk and will help prevent or reduce the severity, frequency, and duration of hot flashes. Healthy lifestyle habits are a necessity for menopausal transition and will make for a less erratic brain neuroregulation. Exercise and routine activity, breathwork, relaxation techniques, stress reduction, meditation, balanced work and rest habits, and adequate rest are all proven measures. Finally, avoiding hot drinks, caffeine, alcohol, spicy foods, sugar, environmental and chemical triggers, heat and humidity, and undue stressors will help.

Chapter 3

Hot Flashes— Classical Chinese- Medicine Theory

Classical Chinese Medicine

Classical Chinese medicine is the foundation for the modern practice of acupuncture and Chinese medicine. Though the commentaries on hot flashes and menopausal transition in the classics are minimal, there is a wealth of general knowledge and clues that we, as practitioners, can adapt and introduce into our current medical system to help better understand and treat them.

As previously discussed, there are many classical theories that inform our understanding of the modern hot-flash environment, including concepts related to the zangfu organs, especially the heart and kidney, "chao re," "ministerial fire," "kidney fire," "heart fire," and "yin fire."

The following passages from chosen classics provide a great deal of insight.

Understanding these classical medical concepts are the vital components that today's acupuncture and Chinese medical practitioners need to know to build a solid foundation for treating the modern hot flash.

Shang Han Lun

In the *Shang Han Lun* 伤寒论 (*Treatise on Cold Damage*), written by Zhang Zhong Jing (150–219 CE), there are more than 20 references to "chao re" 潮热 and "tidal heat effusion." These references from the *Shang Han Lun* emphasize one major hot-flash concept—that tidal heat effusion is the result of internal heat repletion and stagnation issues located primarily in the yangming and shaoyang. Heat repletion can consume and dry out the yin, creating yin vacuity heat signs including tidal heat/fever, night sweats, constipation, etc. Addressing and treating repletion patterns is warranted in the treatment of some hot-flash patients by utilizing acupuncture and herbal formulas that purge heat and regulate qi.

One of the principal formulas from the *Shang Han Lun* to treat chao re is Da Cheng Qi Tang, which is primarily used to purge accumulated heat. In the modern clinic, this formula is commonly known as a constipation formula. This, however, is a narrow viewpoint and can lead practitioners to believe that if there are no significant constipation issues, the formula is unwarranted and may purge vital qi and harm the patient by stimulating excessive bowel movements, leading to diarrhea and general spleen qi deficiency symptoms.

This formula is very effective for treating excess heat stagnation and for healing a wide variety of symptoms, not just constipation. It is true that heat can injure the fluids, making them viscous and turbid, and drying out the stool, causing severe constipation and frequent gas. Heat stagnation can also generate tidal fever symptoms much like hot flashes, resulting from injured yin, yangming heat disease at 3–5pm (heat steaming the body fluids), focal distension in the three jiao, sweating of the hands and feet, a prickled tongue with a yellow, dry coating, and a deep and forceful pulse. Other symptoms to be aware of are skin rashes, stress or irritability, swelling, or other irregular and accompanying symptoms that fit the overall pattern.

This is just one of many hot-flash environment patterns. It can often be seen in younger women, perhaps in their thirties and forties, and in women during the perimenopause who believe they are entering early menopause.

Tidal heat effusion is classically due to patients of all ages getting sick from a cold or flu, which then makes its way further inwards, causing stagnation and heat repletion. This pattern is not exclusive to women; it can be seen in male patients as well. As I understand it, this pattern can also be the result of long-standing emotional stresses on the body, irregular dietary habits that are not suited to the person's body, or other pathologies that lead to this excess pattern. The reason this is an important concept to understand is that tidal heat effusions of this sort are not typical hot flashes due to menopause, but are the result of an internal excess heat stagnation pattern. If this pattern occurs in conjunction with menopausal transition, the hot flashes will be more intense, severe, constant, and sometimes intractable to treatment.

The following lines from the *Shang Han Lun—On Cold Damage Translation & Commentaries* provide fresh and valuable insight, strengthening our clinical diagnostic skills and general understanding of the excess-type hot-flash environment. The *Shang Han Lun* is one of the greatest Chinese-medicine clinical manuals ever to be written. Keep in mind that the provided quotations are only portions of a much larger context and commentary.

Line 137 and Commentary

> A feeling of heat that occurs at set intervals and may or may not be accompanied by palpable heat effusion. (Mitchell, Ye, and Wiseman 1998, p.220)

This is a common definition of "chao re" or tidal heat effusion. The heat comes and goes like the waves of the ocean. This can be confusing because the feeling of heat comes and goes at a constant rate. Hot flashes also come and go, but they are not necessarily at regular set intervals. Heat repletion patterns are more consistent.

Line 220 and Commentary

> Tidal heat effusion is the type of heat effusion generally seen in yang brightness patterns... Tidal heat effusion is heat effusion with a set

periodicity which, when associated with yang brightness patterns, is generally said to occur in the late afternoon and early evening, roughly between the hours of 3 p.m. and 7 p.m.—the hours when the qi of the yang brightness is effulgent. (Mitchell, Ye, and Wiseman 1998, p.337)

A yang brightness pattern means the issue is affecting the stomach and large intestine (yangming) jing qi. This is why the clinician should be asking about the patient's digestion. We can also see that heat repletion has the tendency to build up and release in regular intervals, especially in the late afternoon and early evening. Patients in this category will experience hot-flash type symptoms more during this time of day that will subside or disappear entirely for the rest of the day, along with other subsequent symptoms.

Line 209 and Commentary

When in yang brightness disease, [there is] tidal heat effusion and slightly hard stool, one can give Major Qi-Coordinating Decoction (da cheng qi tang)… Yang brightness disease with tidal heat effusion and hard stool. This pattern is yang brightness bowel repletion with exuberant interior dryness-heat and it is treated with Major Qi-Co-ordinating Decoction (da cheng qi tang). (Mitchell, Ye, and Wiseman 1998, pp.358–359)

This entry further emphasizes that the generation of tidal heat is the result of heat stagnation in the yangming or digestive tract. This pattern presents with constipation, tidal fever at dusk, shortness of breath, irritability, thirst, a dry tongue coating, and a full or wiry and forceful pulse. One of the chief diagnostic questions the clinician should ask is if there is a history of constipation or difficulty with the bowel movements. If present, the practitioner must address this first in order to treat the hot flashes. If the patient's stools are not appropriately addressed, relieving hot flashes in the traditional sense of addressing the kidney may only provide mild or temporary relief.

Line 214 and Commentary

> When in yang brightness disease [there is] delirious speech, tidal heat effusion, and a pulse that is slippery and racing. (Mitchell, Ye, and Wiseman 1998, p.334)

In the clinic, it's possible for a hot-flash patient to present with a slippery and racing pulse. This usually indicates exuberant heat versus the traditional menopausal-transition hot-flash environment pulse, which is generally weaker, thinner, or slightly rapid. It is a good idea to question the patient regarding an increase in appetite or frequency of eating habits, which may indicate stomach heat. Be aware, though, that this may also be due to stomach yin deficiency rather than excess. Patients with qi deficiency traditionally will not have excessive hunger symptoms but may overeat for other reasons including emotional eating or out of fatigue. Some patients may also present with symptoms of shen or spirit disturbances. It is a good idea when talking with your patient to determine if the patient is focused or easily distracted and whether they have any sleep issues.

Line 137 and Commentary

> When in greater yang disease, sweating is promoted repeatedly, yet precipitation is [also used] and [there is] inability to defecate for five or six days, a dry tongue and thirst, minor tidal heat effusion in the late afternoon, and hardness, fullness, and pain, [extending] from below the heart to the lesser abdomen and [which the person will] not allow [anyone even to get] near, Major Chest Bind Decoction (da xian xiong tang) governs... Tidal heat effusion occurs in bowel repletion and is not generally mild, as it is here. (Mitchell, Ye, and Wiseman 1998, p.220)

From time to time, a patient may present with hot flashes that started relatively soon after being sick with a cold or flu, or with the above-mentioned accompanying pain symptoms in the chest and diaphragm. Heat repletion and stagnation in the chest and diaphragm or in the digestive tract can both generate hot flashes, but the main difference is the location of the pronounced discomfort. Pain in the chest, diaphragm, and abdomen is commonly the result of a relatively acute qi stagnation pattern, whether due to stress and emotional upset or dietary issues. Qi stagnation does not allow the water metabolism to move freely, which generates fullness and hardness of the epigastrium or entire abdomen, causing severe pain that is worse with pressure. Relieving the excessive stagnation in the chest and diaphragm by treating the yangming and shaoyang jing qi will ameliorate the hot flashes.

Lines 231 and 104 and Commentary

Shortness of breath, fullness of the entire abdomen, [and] pain under the rib-side and in the heart, which [gives rise to] qi blockage when pressed for a long time, dry nose, inability to sweat, somnolence, yellowing of the entire body including the eyes, difficult urination, tidal heat effusion, frequent hiccup, and swelling in front of and behind the ear. When needling [brings] slight recovery, [but] the exterior has not resolved, [and] the disease has [lasted] more than ten days and the pulse is still floating, one should give Minor Bupleurum Decoction (xiao chai hu tang). (Mitchell, Ye, and Wiseman 1998, pp.396–397)

Fullness in the chest and rib-side, retching, late afternoon tidal heat effusion, and shortly afterward mild diarrhea. This was originally a [Major] Bupleurum [Decoction] (da chai hu tang) pattern... Tidal heat effusion means repletion. It is appropriate to first take Minor Bupleurum Decoction (xiao chai hu tang) in order to resolve the external [aspect]. (Mitchell, Ye, and Wiseman 1998, p.435)

These quotations further illuminate qi stagnation or "blockage" of the yang channels, primarily the shaoyang jing qi, suggesting perhaps a stubborn or chronic disorder. Some hot-flash patients will present with various stubborn or chronic symptoms that have eluded effective relief during previous treatments. Shaoyang is known for its chronicity and is often due to an excess/deficiency situation. The beautiful nature of Chinese medicine is its amazing effectiveness in treating these conditions by reducing the excess qi stagnation or heat repletion and simultaneously nourishing the deficiencies in the blood, yin, qi, and yang.

Line 208 and Commentary

> If [there is] copious sweating, mild heat effusion and aversion to cold, the exterior has not yet resolved, [and given that] this heat [effusion] is not tidal. (Mitchell, Ye, and Wiseman 1998, p.357)

Daytime sweating, especially spontaneous sweating or larger and continuous amounts of sweating, are not typical symptoms of menopausal transition but signs of heat repletion and/or qi deficiency. As the quotation states, the heat is not tidal but mild, meaning that it is low-grade and constant in nature. Traditionally, during menopausal transition, the heat will ebb and flow along with the yin and yang. Consistent heat, on the other hand, is due to either a more severe yin depletion or one of heat repletion. It is natural for typical hot-flash patients to concurrently present with sweating issues, particularly night sweating directly following rushes of heat. It is also common for menopausal-transition patients to have problems of qi deficiency and spontaneous sweats or heat repletion generating sweat. It is also natural for some of these patients to feel warm or hot all of the time. If this happens at a younger age, it is more commonly due to an excess condition, while at a later age like post-menopause, it is more likely due to yin depletion or an excess/deficient heat scenario. Resolving the source of heat and consolidating the exterior will quell the feelings of warmth and stop the sweating.

Nan Jing

Combing through the classical Chinese medical texts in the search for supporting evidence is a laborious task and it may feel as if one is looking for needles in haystacks. The *Huangdi Bashiyi Nan Jing* 黄帝八十一难经 (*The Yellow Emperor's Canon of Eighty-One Difficult Issues*), written in the early Han Dynasty, holds one particular key of importance, found within the text of the Eleventh Difficult Issue, to understanding the hot-flash environment.

The Eleventh Difficult Issue

(1) The scripture states: If the movement in the vessels stops once in less than fifty [arrivals], this is because one long-term depot is void of qi. Which long-term depot is it? (2) It is like this. [The qi] a person inhales enter [the organism] through yin [long-term depots; the qi a person] exhales leave [the organism] through yang [long-term depots. (3) In this case] now, [the qi] inhaled cannot reach the kidneys; they return after they have reached the liver. Hence, the long-term depots which will be void of qi are, obviously, the kidneys; their qi will be depleted first. (Unschuld 2016b, p.130)

This entry addresses the issue at the heart of many age-related health problems in today's modern world, including the hot flash and other menopausal-transition symptoms.

It starts by saying that one of the zangfu organs (depot) will be void of qi (or cut off from the rest) if there is a problem with the flow of qi in the vessels. This references the flow of qi and blood within the daily 24-hour yin and yang cycle. The entry continues by stating that this cycle is directly linked to the inhalation (via the yin organs) and exhalation (via the yang organs), presumably directly referencing how the breath and respiration are governed by the communication between the lung and kidney qi.

Here is the crucial element: the text goes on to say that if there is a problem with this mechanism, over time the qi will only reach the level of the liver before returning to the lung. The kidney, then void of qi, will be cut off from receiving qi from the zangfu organs, leading to its depletion.

What is quite remarkable about this *Nan Jing* entry is that it highlights the importance of cause and effect. First, if the flow of yin and yang is disturbed, there will be dysfunction. Second, it directly links the flow of qi and blood to the breath. If the breath is in dysfunction, it will cause problems for the vessels. Third, it links the dysfunction of the vessels to the decline of the zangfu organs, mainly and starting with the kidney. The evidence leads to the conclusion that in order to maintain the internal health of the zangfu organs, one must maintain proper health of the respiration.

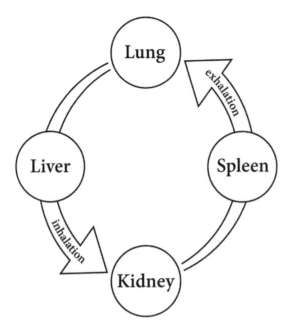

Lung-kidney connection

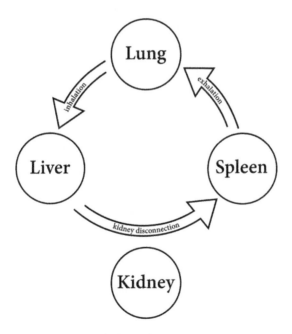

Lung-kidney disconnection

FIGURE 3.1: LUNG AND KIDNEY—QI DISCONNECTION

This raises two important factors about the aging process and our modern lifestyle. First, it is natural to become less active as we age, but with less activity, the lung and kidney will slowly lose their strength and qi communication. Second, in our industrialized society, we are naturally more inclined to a sedentary lifestyle (or have lost our physical, mental, and spiritual focus), again weakening the qi communication between the lung and kidney. This directly affects the flow of qi and blood and the eventual weakening of the zangfu organs and their ability to generate qi.

Once this cycle is established, the inevitable conclusion is that the kidney becomes cut off (void of qi) and begins to decline. Chinese-medicine theory regularly discusses the gradual decline of the kidney during the aging process, including the kidney yin, yang, and essence. What is fascinating, though, is this particular entry suggests the individual plays an active role in this process. Our lifestyle habits have a direct impact on the overall aging process, including menopausal transition.

Traditionally, we talk about the kidney and liver when discussing menopausal transition and the hot-flash environment. This *Nan Jing* entry provides a vital component in explaining the hot flash. For example, use the common pattern of kidney yin with exuberant yang qi to explain the hot flash. This entry states that the kidney is void of qi, meaning it is cut off from receiving qi from above. It slowly goes into decline and is unable to supply yin (water) to balance the liver yang and to quell the heart fire. The other issue is that once the kidney is not in communication with the lung, the lung-spleen-kidney axis will lose its ability to generate new qi, creating further issues. This skips the vital flow of qi down to the kidney and then back up through the spleen and to the lung. Although not confirmed in the text, it is probable that the dysregulation throws off the lung-spleen-kidney axis in manufacturing and supplying yuan qi to the body, further exacerbating yang qi, weakening yin, and diminishing the manufacturing process of qi, thus depleting qi and blood.

The final piece of the puzzle: when the lung cannot descend, it loses its qi connection with the kidney and the liver becomes overactive.

The ascending nature of the liver becomes exaggerated and the lung becomes exuberant with qi. The dispersing action of the lung becomes overactive, creating continuous dispersion and sweating. Finally, qi eventually becomes exuberant within the upper jiao and harasses the spirit and agitates heart fire.

The qi from the lung descends and stops at the liver. The liver is the regulator of yin and yang and the movement of qi. If the liver begins receiving the yang from above and cannot pass it down into the kidney, it will inevitably become overpowered by yang qi. The liver will then be imbalanced and its yin will decline in two ways: by not communicating with and receiving yin from the kidney and by becoming effulgent in yang qi from above. The effect will be an excess of yang qi rising back up from the liver and harassing the heart, resulting in heart fire and the hot-flash environment.

This *Nan Jing* entry confirms that in order to treat this situation, it is necessary to reestablish the kidney's qi communication with the lung and the rest of the zangfu organs.

Clinically, one could make the argument that it is necessary to nourish the kidney since they are cut off and being depleted. But this is like airdropping food and first-aid supplies to a nation cut off from the rest of the world: it may provide some temporary improvement but is not a solution. This is reminiscent of either prescribing kidney tonics in the Chinese medical clinics or prescribing hormone-replacement therapies in the Western medical clinics. It is only a solution for the symptom, not the solution for the underlying problem.

The proper and long-term solution is to reconnect the kidney to the rest of the zangfu organs, much like reestablishing the ground supply chain to the cut-off nation. In the Chinese medical clinic, this means reestablishing the kidney and lung qi communication and regaining control of the respiration. Once this happens, the yin and yang will become balanced and the qi and blood will flow freely through the channels. I liken this to establishing a new flow of healthy blood throughout the body, balancing yin and yang, and, ultimately, effectively treating the hot-flash environment. The healthier the body, the less evident and problematic the hot flashes.

Pi Wei Lun

In the *Pi Wei Lun* 脾胃论 (*Treatise of the Spleen and Stomach*), Li Dong Yuan (1180–1252 CE) supports the theories that stomach qi is the root of humans and the stomach is the sea of the five viscera and six bowels; its clear qi pours upward into the lung. The water and grains we consume enter the stomach, the stomach floats the essence qi to the spleen, the spleen spreads the essence, the essence gathers in the lung, the lung opens the flow of water passages, and finally water fluids are transported down to the urinary bladder. The water and essence ultimately spreads in the four directions and to the five channels. It runs side by side with the four seasons and five viscera, and the measurements of yin and yang. Thus normalcy is kept.

In the chapter "Treatise on Initiation of Heat in the Center Due to Damage by Food & Drink and Taxation Fatigue," Li Dong Yuan further supports the theory that the spleen and stomach are at the center of the body and zangfu organ system. Dietary irregularities, immoderate eating, or the seven affects (joy, anger, anxiety, thought, sorrow, fear, and fright) will damage the spleen, stomach, and yuan qi. Damage to the center qi pours downwards and disrupts and causes the ministerial fire to counterflow upwards and accumulate in the heart, thus generating heart fire or yin fire. The *Pi Wei Lun* states: "If the spleen and stomach qi become decrepit and original qi becomes insufficient, heart fire becomes effulgent on its own. This heart fire is a yin fire. It starts from the lower burner and its ligation links to the heart" (Flaws 2007, p.81).

The crux of the argument is that when spleen qi becomes deficient, heart fire becomes exuberant. Weak spleen and stomach qi pours downward into the mingmen (life gate), accumulates, and stirs the ministerial fire. Frenetic ministerial fire counterflows upwards along the kidney channel linking with the pericardium to accumulate in the heart.

Symptoms of yin fire include raised qi with dyspnea, generalized fever, vexation, large or surging pulse, headache, thirst, aversion to wind (cold and heat) with alternating hot and cold, and surging pulse that is floating, slippery, and forceful. This is a true excess/deficiency pattern. Perimenopause, menopausal transition, and post-menopause patients alike can commonly present with these symptoms.

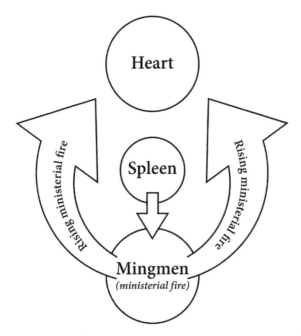

FIGURE 3.2: *PI WEI LUN*—GENERATION OF MINISTERIAL FIRE

Li Dong Yuan provides the classic herbal formula for spleen and stomach qi deficiency—Bu Zhong Yi Qi Tang 补中益气汤 (Tonify the Middle and Augment the Qi Decoction). The entire *Pi Wei Lun* is based on this hallmark and foundational formula. It is classically known for treating low-grade heat manifestations due to qi deficiency. Its actions are to tonify the qi of the middle jiao and raise sunken yang, thus supporting the qi of the spleen and stomach.

There are five traditional disease mechanisms that give rise to yin fire, or the pathological upward stirring of ministerial fire, thus causing hot flashes. They include spleen qi deficiency, liver depression, damp-heat, yin and blood deficiency, and stirring of ministerial fire.

Spleen Qi Deficiency

Spleen qi deficiency is a common pattern seen in the clinic, no matter what the patient's complaint, and is largely due to living in our modern society. The main causes of this pattern are: psychological and emotional issues such as overthinking, anxiety, or worry; physical issues such as over-exercising, working long hours, or a sedentary lifestyle; poor dietary habits; or incorrect medical treatments, including herbs, vitamins, or supplements that damage the spleen.

Once the spleen has been damaged, this is called spleen qi deficiency because the spleen cannot work optimally. It cannot perform its job of moving and transforming water, and this leads to water gathering, accumulating, and transforming into dampness. This accumulated dampness can obstruct the free flow of the yang qi, where it becomes depressed and transforms into depressed heat. Depressed heat can combine with the already accumulated dampness, forming damp-heat that can pour downwards into the lower jiao. The end result is damp-heat harassing and agitating the ministerial fire, causing it to flare upwards and resulting in hot flashes.

Damage to the spleen will also affect its ability to generate new blood, leading to blood deficiency. As previously discussed, blood regeneration is vital to a woman's health and healthy blood is necessary to help control hot flashes. When blood is deficient, the yin will also be affected, leading to difficulty controlling yang. Unchecked yang, as previously discussed, not only has the tendency to ascend, but can stir the ministerial fire as well, generating hyperactive fire.

The problem with spleen qi deficiency is that it weakens the entire system from multiple angles, meaning the longer it is left untreated, the more problematic it is. Treatment of this scenario includes targeting the source issue by tonifying the spleen and removing the underlying causes of the spleen qi deficiency.

Liver Depression

Liver depression, also known as liver qi stagnation in Chinese medicine, means that the liver's ability to maintain the smooth movement of qi throughout the body is compromised, resulting in qi stagnation. The primary causes of liver depression are unfulfilled desires, anger issues, physical or mental fatigue, and dietary habits rich in spice, grease, processed foods, or alcohol. The liver can lose its ability to regulate qi and keep the physiological functions of the body running smoothly. Liver depression leads to stagnant qi, and stagnant qi, once constrained over time, develops into heat stagnation. Stagnated heat has the tendency to rise and harass the heart. It can also follow deficiency qi and dampness downwards, gather in the lower jiao, and harass the ministerial fire, which in turn will flare upwards, also harassing the heart and creating hot flashes.

Liver depression is commonly seen in conjunction with spleen qi deficiency in the clinical setting. This is known as an excess/deficiency scenario where the liver (wood) is stronger than and overacts on the spleen (earth), resulting in an imbalance of the two—middle jiao disharmony. This becomes increasingly problematic since the weak spleen qi will continue to sink and stir the ministerial fire, while the overactive liver will continue to stoke the ministerial fire, helping it ascend and harass the heart even further. Finally, as the weakened spleen fails to generate new blood, the liver, which needs new blood to function and store, will become blood deficient and further worsen the situation. Treatment of liver depression needs to focus on smoothing the free flow of its qi, while at the same time addressing the liver yin and yang and remedying the underlying causes.

Damp-Heat

There are three prime causes of a damp-heat issue. The first, as previously described, is the end product of a weakened spleen. The second cause is poor food choices or overeating habits. Over time, sweets, dairy, and grains will engender fluids. Hot and spicy foods and alcohol will engender heat. Greasy, fatty, oily foods will engender dampness. Finally, damp, humid, and hot environments or weather can generate damp-heat in the body. While spleen qi deficiency may take a longer time frame to engender damp-heat, dietary choices and the environment can have a fast and dramatic effect on the body. The patient's dietary choices, and to a lesser degree their environment, can act as the fuel for the hot-flash fire. Treatment needs to focus on draining damp-heat and helping the patient identify and correct poor diet and environmental issues.

Yin and Blood Deficiency

Yin and blood are constantly being utilized, consumed, and regenerated in women. As mentioned, these have the tendency to become increasingly deficient as women age. Yin and blood anchor yang qi and quell fire. Without their abundance, the tendency for hot flashes increases during menopausal transition. Treatment for yin and blood deficiency is primarily through tonifying herbal formulas and good nutrition, along with a balanced daily life routine. It is vital for women to eat well and maintain a healthy emotional environment to balance the liver and support the spleen, and to keep active and find time to rest to support and balance the heart, lung, and kidney.

Stirring of Ministerial Fire

There are several factors that can generate the stirring of ministerial fire. The direct stoking and strengthening of yang qi within the mingmen creates this pattern. Puberty, excessive libido, recreational drugs, and excessive mental activity all have the tendency to directly stimulate and increase the yang qi to stir the ministerial fire. This is not uncommon, and some hot-flash patients will clinically present only with stirring of the ministerial fire. It is necessary to question the patient to identify possible causes. Treatment is often centered on anchoring yang qi, draining damp-heat, quelling fire, and calming the spirit.

Conclusion

All five patterns have the tendency to stir the ministerial fire and generate hot flashes, at any age in life, in children and men alike. The key takeaway for the practitioner is to understand how these patterns play out in the course of a woman's health history leading up to menopausal transition.

The Fire Spirit School

Theories from the Fire Spirit School offer new insight into the hot-flash environment. Traditionally, in Chinese medicine, the hot flash is considered to be the rising of an unabated (yang) fire leaping away from a deficient (yin) water source. The treatment is to supplement yin and to descend the fire. In contrast, Zheng Qinan 鄭欽安 (1804–1901 CE) describes an alternative strategy: leading the unabated fire back to the lower source within the mingmen. The theory is to reestablish the balance of yin and yang by supporting the true yang below.

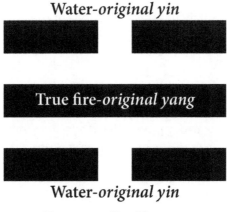

Water-*original yin*

True fire-*original yang*

Water-*original yin*

FIGURE 3.3: KAN TRIGRAM

The theory of the Fire Spirit School starts with the understanding that the original or true yang resides within the original or true yin. This is based on the Kan trigram (I Ching), where one fire is found between one water above and one water below. The mingmen fire, or true yang, residing between the two kidneys (water) reflects this idea. This is where the true yang (fire) generates yin (water). Together, the two balance and control one another.

Hot flashes are not traditionally considered the result of the excessive rising of true yang. Hot flashes are normally considered an empty heat ascending from a deficient yin source. Zheng Qinan provides us with a unique perspective as the following doctrine states:

> …empty fire rushes upwards, it clearly binds with the surging water (water is Yin). If the water surges one fraction, the dragon surges as well one fraction (dragon is fire). If the water is higher one foot then the dragon is higher one foot as well. The dragon is roaming because the water is surging. It is not that the dragon fails to dive and acts

contrary to its normal state. Therefore the classic states: When the Yin surges the Yang must decline. One can realize that by the application of medicinals one must support the Yang and restrain the Yin. (Seidman and Ming 2011, Scroll One, p.18)

There are two important concepts presented. First, surging yin (excess) is due to deficient yang. The true yang within the yin will inevitably rise, along with the surging yin. Second, the treatment in this situation is to use yang medicinals. The idea is to lead the fire downwards and back to the source by fortifying the true yang, thus restraining surging yin. It goes on to say:

Kan functions normally when original Yang, the true fire, burns at the bottom. When Yin surges, original Yang leaves the bottom position and burns at the wrong places. That is why fire syndrome can occur in Yin syndrome. (Seidman and Ming 2011, Scroll One, p.19)

Here, Zheng Qinan clearly explains a hot-flash scenario. When the true yang rises with the surging yin, it "burns at the wrong places." This means the true yang burns in the heart and upper portions of the body. This is an excess yin and not a deficient yin pattern. The fire is not in excess; it is merely in the wrong location.

This is a common hot-flash presentation in the clinic. It looks similar to exuberant ministerial fire or damp-heat accumulation. The patient presents with a rapid, forceful, or surging pulse, along with an exuberance of excess yin and fire symptoms. The first response as a practitioner may be to subdue the yang, quell the fire, and induce diuresis to drain the excess yin. However, with further analysis, the patient's situation is an excess yin with deficient fire presentations. Zheng Qinan explains:

Even though on the surface fire symptoms are apparent (this fire is called empty/deficient fire and is different than full/excess fire. Excess fire results from guest energy entering Yang channels and oppressing them. Deficient fire takes place when Yin Qi rises to overstep its authority. Yin means water, while Qi is the pre-heaven Yang within the water and therefore it is named deficient fire. When water's energy flows downward it is suitable and when upward it is inappropriate. It is truly because the emperor fire is too weak and can't calmly receive it, resulting in the upward overstepping and the disease), they resemble excess fire. (Seidman and Ming 2011, Scroll One, pp.39–40)

The fire is deemed deficient in nature but is not the product of a yin deficiency pattern. Therefore, quelling and draining fire is unwarranted. As mentioned earlier, to treat this pattern, it is necessary to lead the fire back to the source with yang medicinals. "When fire is vigorous then Yin disappears on its own. It is like the strong sun that scatters the clouds until they disappear" (Seidman and Ming 2011, Scroll One, p.18). Yin and yang will be balanced when the true yang is fortified.

This hot-flash environment is created by chronic, abnormal, or excessive lifestyle habits including diet, taxation, and unchecked emotions. When the practitioner takes a closer look, they will see that the patient suffers from fatigue and other qi and yang deficiency symptoms.

Fu Qing Zhu Gynecology

The famous gynecology Chinese-medicine doctor Fu Qing Zhu (1607–1684 CE) incorporated his wisdom into his book *Fu Qing Zhu Nu Ke* 傅青主女科 (*Women's Diseases According to Fu Qing-Zhu*). The following quotes highlight his wisdom and further support proper diagnosis and treatment of "True Fire," "Kidney Fire," and "Fire Qi" patterns, thus addressing hot flashes. What is most interesting and helpful is that Fu Qing Zhu leads us through a deeper understanding of a woman's potential excess and deficiency environment and how to treat the imbalances of yin and yang based on the understanding.

First Quote

When fire is too effulgent, blood gets hot. When water is too effulgent, the blood becomes abundant... It is true that superabundant fire cannot be left unattended, but in no circumstances should water be made insufficient. Therefore, the treatment method is just to clear a little without draining water. (Yang and Liu 2010, pp.29–30)

This first quote is amazing and gives us guidance for treating hot flashes in women who have a relatively excess hot-flash environment. The yang qi is abundant and the yin qi is relatively intact. There are many hot-flash patients in perimenopause, menopausal transition, and post-menopause that will have this presentation. These patients commonly have a full and forceful pulse and heat symptoms, and are generally active and boisterous. It is an excess heat pattern. Fu Qing Zhu recommends using the formula Qing Jing San to eliminate heat, prevent injury to yin, and cool the blood. This quote was originally used for treating women with early menstrual cycles.

Qing Jing San 清经散 (Clear the Menses Powder): Mu dan pi, di gu pi, bai shao, shu di huang, qing hao, fu ling, huang bai.

Second Quote

> …extreme hot blood. Who would suspect effulgent fire in the kidneys with depletion of yin water? And, why should there be one classification of vacuity and another of repletion… (In this case,) the treatment method is to exclusively supplement water without draining fire. Once water becomes abundant, fire is automatically extinguished. (Yang and Liu 2010, pp.30–31)

This second quote is similar to the first, with a presentation of excess yang qi, but the difference is that the yin qi is damaged. This is a common hot-flash presentation, one of excess yang and deficiency of yin. Fu Qing Zhu recommends that the practitioner does not take the bait and try to clear fire, but supplements water to bring balance back to yin and yang, thus quelling the hot flash with the formula Liang Di Tang. This formula nourishes blood and supplements water without draining fire. Once water becomes effulgent, fire is naturally extinguished and rectified. His original indication was for treating early and heavy menses due to blood deficiency and raging fire qi.

Liang Di Tang 两地汤 (Rehmannia and Lycium Root Bark Decoction): Sheng di huang, xuan shen, bai shao, mai men dong, di gu pi, e jiao.

Third Quote

> Blood is yin. When blood becomes vacuous, yang must become hyperactive. Hyperactivity (of yang) does harm…whereas fire is burning ragingly, yin water cannot be engendered quickly enough for the transformation of blood. As a result, (kidney) yin becomes vacuous and fire is stirred… (However,) this fire is a vacuity fire. Replete fire allows for drainage, but vacuity fire requires clearing by way of supplementation. In this way, vacuity fire is easy to dissipate and true fire will be engendered… If stomach yang stops being engendered, what else can transform the refined essence to engender yin water? (Yang and Liu 2010, pp.83–84)

This is a fascinating and lengthy train of thought. Fu Qing Zhu takes us into the understanding of how deficiency of yin creates the relative yang qi excess environment. What is interesting here is the idea that once fire becomes excessive due to the deficiency of yin (which can happen naturally in women), the newly generated fire halts the natural ability of the body to generate new yin, thus creating a vicious excess/deficiency cycle. He suggests supplementation in order to maintain the ability to generate new yin by protecting the true fire, which is the yang qi. This is along the same lines as Li Dong Yuan's theory of supporting the middle qi to treat disease. In today's modern society, it is very easy to see this situation where the body cannot generate fresh yin and blood because the spleen and stomach qi are weak. The relative fire is to be controlled and not to be purged. He recommends the formula Jia Jian Si Wu Tang to help engender yin and blood, cool the yang within the blood, and support the spleen and stomach to generate new yin.

Jia Jian Si Wu Tang 加减四物汤 (Modified Four Herb Decoction): Shu di huang, bai shao, dang gui, chuan xiong, (+) zhi zi, shan zhu yu, shan yao, mu dan pi.

Fourth Quote

> People all declare (this due to) extremely exuberant fire, but do they know in which channel this fire is so effulgent? …but fire, if excessive,

will dry up water... Suppose the fire in the stomach is over-effulgent. This will inevitably dry up kidney water... When earth is burning extremely intensely, the blazing flames gain such momentum that they invade the heart and trespass against the spirit... Disease in the second yang (i.e. yang ming) expands to the heart and spleen. (Yang and Liu 2010, pp.73–74)

This quote is important to understand in treating hot flashes because it plainly explains how yangming (stomach), which sits just below the heart, when filled with yang qi or heat, can rise and harass the heart. As discussed, the heart is at the center of the hot-flash environment, and if heart fire is generated, the hot flash can be too. There are many patients who may present with other common patterns for hot flashes who will also have concurrent dueling patterns such as yangming excess. This excess is commonly seen with our modern dietary choices, overeating, and overindulgences. We eat out of stress, out of habit, and for comfort, and it is easy for these eating habits to generate yangming excess. This quote was written originally for the same pattern causing possible miscarriages in women. Even though there may be more suitable formulas, the takeaway here is the importance of draining the stomach fire to calm the heart fire. Fu Qing Zhu recommends the formula Xi Fen An Tai Tang to drain fire, enrich water, and calm the shen.

Xi Fen An Tai Tang 息焚安胎汤 (Quench the Conflagration and Calm the Fetus Decoction): Sheng di huang, qing hao, bai zhu, fu ling, ren shen, zhi mu, tian hua fen.

Fifth Quote

...qi and blood are seriously depleted and it is natural that kidney water is insufficient and that kidney fire is boisterous. Water, when insufficient, is unable to nurture the liver... However, this effulgent fire of liver/wood is only a false appearance. This fire is not really effulgent. Falsely effulgent qi seems exuberant, but, in fact, it is insufficient. Therefore, sometimes there occurs fever and sometimes cold... This cold is not true cold; this heat is not true heat. They are (manifestations of) unsoothed qi due to counterflow between the chest and diaphragm… The appropriate treatment method is to supplement the blood to nurture the liver and supplement the essence to engender the blood. (Yang and Liu 2010, p.125)

This is a wonderful example of the complexities due to a long-standing yin and yang imbalance. What is presented is the continued taxation of the yin and blood (water) of the body, resulting in yang (fire) excess. This is a normal menopausal transition and post-menopause presentation that also can be more difficult to treat. What Fu Qing Zhu explains here is the development of the liver's role in this scenario. He clearly points out how difficult it can be to manage qi and blood flow and regulate body temperature within this environment.

Many practitioners know that menopausal-transition patients experience the fluctuations of hot and cold feelings. This is due to the yin deficiency being unable to harness the yang and unable to "nurture" the liver. As we know, the liver and kidney share the same source, so when the kidney is injured, it will eventually affect the liver. Along with the difficulty in body temperature regulation, we also see an interesting situation where the liver then cannot regulate the smooth flow of qi, which in turn creates stagnation in the chest and diaphragm. Once this is established, women will have difficulty maintaining emotional balance, there will be stomach and digestive issues, and they will have difficulty managing their breathing. These will create even more issues for the heart, which will already have been harassed by its imbalance with the kidney. The recommended formula is Zhuan Qi Tang, which supplements the essence and blood. As you see again, and further supporting the argument to always treat the blood in menopausal transition, Fu Qing Zhu doesn't recommend draining fire or even moving qi but nourishing the blood and essence.

Zhuan Qi Tang 转气汤 (Change the Qi Decoction): Ren shen, fu ling, bai zhu, dang gui, bai shao, shu di huang, shan zhu yu, shan yao, qian shi, chai hu, gu zhi.

Sixth Quote

> But when hot evils exist in the precincts of the lower burner, fluids are
> no longer able to transform into essence but transform (instead) into
> dampness. Dampness, the qi of earth, is, practically (speaking), the
> intrusion of water. While heat, the qi of fire, is, practically (speaking),
> engendered by wood... How can it be cured by merely attending to the
> spleen? The appropriate method is to supplement conception vessel
> vacuity and to clear flaming kidney fire. (Yang and Liu 2010, p.8)

This essential quotation presents a damp-heat accumulation in the
lower jiao scenario. Fu Qing Zhu clearly explains how dampness accumulation interferes with the engenderment of yin and essence and
the subsequent buildup of qi and heat, resulting in damp-heat accumulation. Chinese-medicine practitioners understand that dampness
is the result of a weakened spleen qi, but he questions the efficacy of
treatment based solely on engendering the spleen.

His recommended formula is Yi Huang Tang, which is a traditional
formula to drain damp-heat in the lower jiao with the symptoms of
leucorrhea. Most women do not experience leucorrhea issues during
menopausal transition. Nonetheless, some will present with damp-heat
accumulation. As we see with this citation, this plays into the hot-flash
environment perfectly by adding additional stress to an already present
yin and essence deficiency. Many women will present in the clinic with
difficult and intractable hot flashes due to this situation. This formula
clears the kidney fire and resolves heat. Chronic dampness cannot be
given a way out unless kidney fire is cleared.

Yi Huang Tang 易黄汤 (Change Yellow (Discharge) Decoction): Chao
shan yao, chao qian shi, huang bai, che qian zi, bai guo.

Seventh Quote

> The *Za Zheng Lun (The Treatise on Miscellaneous Conditions)* says,
> "Spontaneous sweating (is due to) yang depletion; while thief sweating
> (is due to) yin vacuity."...Only that which (can) regulate the qi and

> blood in addition (to stopping sweating) is appropriate. (Yang and Liu 2010, p.193)

It is appropriate to finish this section of the discussion on hot flashes with a discussion of sweating. Fu Qing Zhu gives us a description and comparison of two types of sweating: one that is due to yang depletion and one that is due to yin vacuity. It is common for women during menopausal transition to experience night sweating (*thief sweating*), along with hot flashes. But upon closer examination, we may find these patients also have spontaneous sweating throughout. Our previous discussions on yin and yang have addressed concepts of how one can affect the other and present simultaneously. Here, Fu Qing Zhu gives us the key, explaining the need to treat and regulate the qi and blood to stop sweating, further supporting the theory that treating the blood is central to balancing the hot-flash environment. The recommended formula is Zhi Han San, which regulates and supplements qi and blood and constrains sweating. It is a basic qi and blood tonic with supplemental herbs to treat sweating.

One final note: additional herbs to clear the heat from the heart (huang lian) and herbs to calm the spirit (mu li and fu xiao mai) are appropriate since the heart governs the sweat and plays a central role in hot flashes.

Zhi Han San 止汗散 (Stop Sweating Powder): Ren shen, dang gui, shu di huang, ma huang gen, huang lian, fu xiao mai, da zao.

Chapter 4

Hot Flashes—Chinese Medicine Meets Western Medicine

Introduction—The Hot Flash

One objective of this book is to provide a deeper understanding of the hot-flash environment. Looking at the Western scientific approach to hot flashes through the lens of Chinese medicine, it is clear there are many similarities between the neuro-endocrine dynamics of Western medicine and the yin and yang dynamics found in Chinese medicine.

Menopausal Transition

The menstrual cycle functions via a complex negative feedback loop of hormones controlled by the HPO axis. Although diminished ovarian reserve is thought to be the predominant event leading to natural menopause, alterations of the central HPO axis with aging are contributing factors.

The disruption to this negative feedback loop happens with age as the ovarian follicle levels naturally decline, producing less estrogen (estradiol), progesterone, and inhibin. This causes hypothalamus gonadotropin-releasing hormone (GnRH) and pituitary-gland follicle-stimulating hormone (FSH) and luteinizing hormone (LH) levels to rise. Anovulation becomes more common, along with ovarian-follicle depletion. Estrogen, inhibin, and progesterone levels decrease.

The negative feedback loop is opened, GnRH is released at maximum frequency and amplitude, and the FSH and LH levels rise to four times greater than in reproductive years.

In a small percentage of women, ovarian reserves decline (ovarian insufficiency) and the menstrual cycle ceases before age 40. Genetic, autoimmune, environmental, infectious, or medical influences may alter ovarian aging, causing premature ovarian failure and "premature menopause." Surgical menopause is discussed later in the chapter.

Resulting factors include vasomotor symptoms (VMS), such as hot flashes and night sweats, which are the most common menopausal-transition complaint in the clinic. Although the pathophysiology is not clear, the hypothalamus, estrogens, and neurotransmitters (norepinephrine and serotonin) play a role in vasomotor dysfunction.

Accompanying menopausal-transition symptoms include: sleep and cognitive dysfunction; psychosocial changes such as mood changes, poor concentration, impaired memory, and depression; cardiovascular disease, congestive heart failure, and stroke; weight gain and fat distribution; lower reproductive tract changes (due to declining estrogen), including vaginal, bladder, and pelvic floor symptoms, dyspareunia, sexual dysfunction, prolapse, dryness, and incontinence; libido changes directly or indirectly due to declining estrogen or by dyspareunia or vaginal dryness.

Chinese-Medicine Pathophysiology

In the Chinese-medicine pathophysiology theory, the kidney qi ascends an independent course through each of the liver, spleen, and lung. From there, each course reaches on to the heart, which has a direct relationship to the brain.

This provides two important details: first, the kidney and brain have a direct connection, mirroring the HPO axis; second, the liver, spleen, and lung are involved in the process. This demonstrates that our emotions, diet, and activity have the potential to interact and impact the neuro-endocrine system and thermoregulation.

It is unknown whether hot flashes develop from one path or from multiple paths in unison. Rather than the old concepts of a single (kidney) or dual (kidney-heart) organ pattern, it is probable that hot flashes are due to the impact of multiple organ systems.

The real scientific and clinical journey is continued investigations into the networking of qi, blood, yin, yang, and essence for a clearer understanding of pattern differentiations. New pattern differentiations will lead to new point combinations and herbal strategies.

We can make the connection between Chinese medicine and Western science understandings of the hot-flash environment by comparing and contrasting yin and yang qi and Chinese-medicine theory with functions of the brain, neuro-endocrine system, and thermoregulation.

The majority of clinical hot flashes are the result of the effulgent yang rising upwards and dispersing outwards. The heat is not a pathogenic heat but merely waves of heat generated by the imbalance of yin and yang. The effulgent yang is a disruption in balance of the internal yin and yang cycle.

The excess yang qi rising upwards and towards the head can theoretically translate as "excessive brain stimulation." Whether it's stress related to overwork or emotional issues, brain activity works at an accelerated rate or in an undisciplined state. This type of environment can disrupt the hypothalamus and its ability to control thermoregulation.

The quality of blood entering the brain, I propose, is another component. Blood is the product of our diet, nutrition, and hydration. If the quality of blood doesn't incorporate the best components to meet neurotransmitter specifications for smooth functioning, this may, over time, lead to early aging and brain issues.

The blood flow to and within the brain will also affect its physiological functions. Common environmental and lifestyle stressors that have an effect on qi and blood circulation can easily disrupt the hypothalamus. If it is true that hot flashes are far more common today than they were in the past due to modern lifestyle and environmental challenges, it is reasonable to believe that hot flashes can be relieved by balancing yin and yang with the right nutrient-rich foods and with proper lifestyle and exercise habits.

Thermoregulation

Core body temperature normally remains within a specific temperature range called the thermoneutral zone. Along with the daily circadian rhythm, the body temperature is regulated by the hypothalamus and stimulated by the nervous system and various hormones, including thyroid, estrogen, and progesterone.

Hot flashes are triggered by core body-temperature elevations acting within a narrowed thermoneutral zone. Hot flashes occur when the core body temperature reaches the upper threshold. Core body temperature then declines, and if the lower threshold is crossed, shivering occurs.

Normal thermoregulation:

Upper threshold = Sweating.

Lower threshold = Shivering.

Neutral zone = Within which major thermoregulatory responses (sweating and shivering) do not occur.

Elevated sympathetic activation contributes to the initiation of hot flashes by narrowing the thermoneutral zone in symptomatic women. Certain biochemical mechanisms act on thermoregulation. Increased brain norepinephrine narrows the thermoneutral zone (yang activity). Estrogen ameliorates and raises the core body temperature and sweating threshold (yin activity).

Hot flashes are caused by many simultaneous processes in the body, including estrogen depletion, thermoregulation disruption, and neurotransmitter dysregulation. This combination has been referred to as "autonomic neurovascular dysregulation." From a Chinese medical perspective, this encompasses the previously discussed qi and blood and yin and yang theories and mechanisms.

HPO Axis

The main components involved in the menstrual cycle are the hypothalamus, pituitary gland, and ovary. These three combine to control the entire menstrual cycle by forming the HPO axis. They signal to and communicate with one another, via a closed-loop negative feedback mechanism, by secreting hormones through the bloodstream. This is the mechanism behind body thermoregulation, and the hypothalamus is at the center of its control.

The HPO axis works much like the heating system in a house. The thermostat tells the system when it should produce heat and when to cool down. The ovary acts as the temperature within the house, the hypothalamus acts as the thermostat, and the pituitary gland (along with the thyroid gland's function of speeding and slowing metabolism) acts as the furnace.

Imagine your house when you first wake up in the morning on a cold day. Now imagine the cold air (ovary) dropping low enough that the house thermostat (hypothalamus) signals the furnace (pituitary gland) to start warming the house. The furnace continues to run until the house has been sufficiently heated (ovary), and then the thermostat (hypothalamus) gets the signal that the house has been sufficiently heated and turns off the furnace (pituitary gland).

This cycle continues every month from menarche to the final menstrual period (FMP), when the reduction of the ovarian reserve and estrogen leads into menopausal transition and the eventual decline of the HPO axis. The primary concern with the decline of the HPO axis is the control of thermoregulation by the hypothalamus. Menopausal transition and the decline of the HPO axis disrupt the hypothalamus's ability to control body temperature.

During menopausal transition, the thermoneutral zone narrows so there is less variability. If the internal heat is high, there are hot flashes, and if it's too low, there is shivering.

For example, when living in a normal environment, an average, comfortable, body thermoneutral zone will have a high range set at 95°F for when you get hot and a low range set at 65°F for when you get cold. During menopausal transition, the high range is reset to 85°F and the low range is reset to 75°F. A normal thermoneutral zone with a 30°F variable drops during menopausal transition to a 10°F variable. This explains why many menopausal-transition women have difficulty with fluctuating temperatures and regulating body temperature.

Why does the hypothalamus lose its ability to control the thermostat? One issue is the decrease of estrogen in the bloodstream and the brain. The hypothalamus is simply conditioned over the years to having more estrogen. This doesn't mean that it requires a specified amount; it has simply adjusted to certain levels.

When ovarian reserve declines and the volume of estrogen drops in the bloodstream, the hypothalamus must continue to function and maintain balance. This can be considered a withdrawal situation. The hypothalamus has to adjust to provide the same functions without the same level of estrogen to trigger them.

The HPO axis operates much like your home heating system, with a continuous negative feedback loop system regulated and stimulated by the hormones. To better understand the process, it is valuable to consider the individual components and hormones.

Ovaries

The two ovaries sit, one on each side of the uterus, in the lower abdomen. Along with the fallopian tubes and female genitalia, they comprise the female reproductive system. According to Chinese medicine, this system is governed by and has a close and intimate relationship to the kidney. The entire female reproductive system and the kidney are primarily considered yin in nature based on their functions and location.

Hypothalamus and Pituitary Gland

The hypothalamus and pituitary gland are both located in the base of the brain. The hypothalamus is considered to be the thermoregulation control center for the body. The pituitary gland is considered to be the master gland of the body. The brain's location in the head holds a yang position in the body. The nervous system as a whole is yang in nature and function.

The brain also has yin attributes, unlike the yang activities of the central nervous system. The brain is considered the sea of marrow in Chinese medicine. Marrow is the product of essence that is supplied by the kidney, which are all aspects of yin. The HPO axis is an elaborate balance of yin and yang qi. Controlling and regulating, it functions much like the liver, commanding qi in Chinese medicine.

Hormones

The ovary releases the following hormones: estrogen, progesterone, inhibin, and testosterone. The hypothalamus releases GnRH, and the pituitary gland releases FSH and LH. Depending on the time of the menstrual cycle and stage of reproductive aging, one or many of these hormones are secreted into the bloodstream. Hormones stimulate another part of the HPO axis, which in turn will secrete a specific hormone right back. This is called a closed-loop negative feedback system. In one sense, we can consider hormones yin in nature since they travel within the blood. They can also be considered yang in nature because of their stimulating functions.

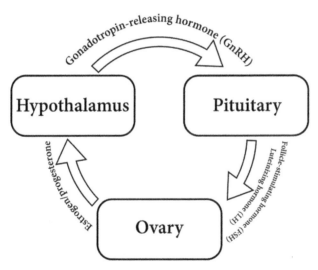

FIGURE 4.1: THE HPO AXIS

The Yin and Yang of the Menstrual Cycle

The HPO axis and hormones establish and synchronize a delicate balance within the body. As a young woman comes into fertility following menarche, the body identifies and grows accustomed to this hormonal balance. The hormones ebb and flow daily and monthly for over 30 years until there is a natural decline in ovarian reserve. While the ovarian reserve slowly diminishes, slow cascades of hormonal changes begin to happen. Some hormones decline and some increase, while others try to maintain synchronicity until they finally settle into their new roles in the postmenopausal era.

During a normal menstrual cycle, the yin and yang dance together. The yin starts out low as low estrogen. The low level of estrogen stimulates the yang component of the cycle. The pituitary gland secretes FSH to increase estrogen. Yang generating yin. As the wellspring of yin gradually increases, so too do the follicle and endometrial lining. Yang continues to generate yin until yin reaches a zenith and explodes. This is ovulation, signaling yang to decline and cool down. Yin and yang wane into rest mode, and then the cycle starts all over again.

Cycles of yin and yang can be seen throughout nature, including in the change of seasons, the cycle of day and night, birth and death, and so on. After 30+ years of this continual menstrual cycle, the yin and yang cycle is disrupted by the decline of ovarian reserve and estrogen.

The pituitary gland must establish a new balance. It is no longer required to produce the same amounts of FSH (yang). At the same time, it is no longer being stimulated by a monthly supply of estrogen (yin) from the ovary. This reestablishment is menopausal transition. It is a rebirth and transformation for all women.

Estrogen

Estrogen is female—it is yin within yin. It is nourishing and gives women their attributes. Estrogen is produced in the ovary and maintains a healthy menstrual cycle, along with help from the hypothalamus and pituitary gland.

There are three types of estrogen produced in the human body. Estrone (E1) is produced during post-menopause by the ovaries, adipose tissue, and adrenal glands. Estradiol (E2) is considered the principal estrogen secreted by the ovaries during reproductive years and the most biologically active in the body. Estriol (E3) is the weakest of the three estrogens and is produced during pregnancy by the placenta.

Estrogen levels begin to rise on day one of the menstrual cycle. This rise signals the pituitary gland to release FSH. This is the natural growth of yin and yang. Estrogen, much like yin, is growth and nutrition. It needs the yang fire of FSH to grow and mature. Estrogen and FSH levels both decrease once ovulation has occurred.

Estrogen has a high expression in the hypothalamus, pituitary gland, adrenal medulla, kidney medulla, and ovary. Estrogen has an effect on the body temperature, blood pressure and cardiovascular system, immune system, mood, metabolism, gastrointestinal tract, sex drive, cognition, mental health, and bone growth and density.

Progesterone

Progesterone is produced and released by the corpus luteum portion of the ovarian follicle. It rises during post-ovulation (yang). Its actions are to provide a steady supply of blood, yin, and essence to the uterine lining for implantation (yin). Progesterone is yang within yin.

Progesterone allows the blood to build within the uterus. Progesterone production drops without fertilization and implantation. The uterine lining sheds and the menstrual period starts.

Supplying qi and blood to the uterus, maintaining continual growth of the lining, preventing contractions, and the release of the uterine lining are all functions that are carried out by the spleen and liver via the chong and ren channels.

Low levels of progesterone have the symptoms of infertility, miscarriage, abnormal uterine bleeding, spotting, and pain. Low progesterone can lead to high levels of estrogen. This is yang deficiency leading to yin excess.

Inhibin

Inhibin is produced by the ovary and regulates the HPO axis. Inhibin A and B have the unique action of starting and stopping the flow of FSH back to the ovary.

During pre-ovulation, Inhibin B is released, which triggers the yang (FSH) to warm the yin (egg). During post-ovulation, Inhibin A is released and inhibits the flow of FSH to the ovary since the egg no longer needs to grow.

Inhibin acts as the temperature gauge. When the house is cold (pre-ovulation), the house thermostat signals the furnace to start warming the house. Here the FSH (yang fire) is helping warm and grow the egg (yin water). When the house is sufficiently heated (post-ovulation), the thermostat turns the furnace off. This illustrates the ovulation process.

FSH and LH

FSH and LH are both produced by the pituitary gland and are the yang counterpart to the ovary and estrogen, which are yin. These two hormones have a true yang within yin function: the FSH provides the continued warmth for the egg to grow, while the strong yang energy of LH stimulates the spark and releases the mature egg.

GnRH

GnRH is produced by the hypothalamus. It is yang in nature and functions to regulate hormone communication and HPO-axis function. The primary goal of GnRH is to stimulate FSH and LH. Testosterone, estrogen, and progesterone (yin) levels control GnRH (yang).

Does Estrogen Deprivation Alone Cause Hot Flashes?

The short answer is no. *Clinical Gynecologic Endocrinology and Infertility—Eighth Edition* states: "Estrogen levels do not begin a major decline until about a year before menopause" (Fritz and Speroff 2011, p.682). Lowered estrogen levels or inappropriately termed "estrogen deficiency syndrome" due to aging have traditionally been regarded as the primary cause of the hot flash. Hot flashes occur in the vast majority of women having natural or surgical menopause. Estrogens are clearly involved in their etiology. This is consistent with the fact that estrogen therapy virtually eliminates hot flashes.

Even though hot flashes do coincide with estrogen withdrawal, it does not entirely explain the phenomenon since estrogen levels do not differ between symptomatic and asymptomatic women:

> Estrogen reduction alone does not explain the occurrence of hot flashes because there are no relationships between these symptoms and plasma, urinary, or vaginal levels of estrogens, nor are there differences in plasma levels between women with and without hot flashes. Additionally, clonidine reduces hot flash frequency but does not change estrogen levels, and prepubertal girls have low estrogen levels but no hot flashes. (Freedman 2014)

Therefore, estrogen decline is a necessary component, but alone it is not sufficient to explain the occurrence of hot flashes. This coincides with the traditional Chinese-medicine view that a drop in estrogen (yin) causes the hot flashes (heat). The question remains however, as to why hot flashes only occur in certain populations.

Estrogen depletion is the removal of a vital component (estrogen) that the body utilized for just under four decades to maintain synchronicity. The brain and the body need to reestablish a new balance. Estrogen is a brain neuromodulator and has an effect on thermoregulation. As serum estrogen levels in the brain decline, this creates a withdrawal scenario that disrupts the ability of the hypothalamus to control body temperature:

> Estrogens are known potent neuromodulators of numerous neuronal circuits throughout the central nervous system. Changing estrogen levels during menopausal transition may impact multiple components involved in maintaining temperature homeostasis. (Deecher and Dorries 2007)

Hypothetically, increased difficulty with reestablishing the balance of the neuro-endocrine system may have its roots in modern lifestyles. It may be affected by consistent brain stimulation, changes in nutrition, and reduced physical activity.

This coincides with societal changes of the past century. Today, in general, we cognitively utilize our brains differently, our work tends to be less physically intensive, and diet and nutrition have been dramatically altered. This has a direct impact on brain neuroregulation, which is directly impacted by stimulation, nutrition, and blood flow within the brain. This affects neuro-endocrine balance and thermoregulation.

Adding estrogen back into the system does alleviate hot flashes in most patients. However, hormone therapy (HT) carries potential and serious health risks.

A small group of women experiencing severe hot flashes do warrant a need for short-term and in rare instances long-term HT treatment. But for most women, the focus should be shifted from utilizing HT as the primary treatment for hot flashes to encouraging significant, concrete, healthy changes in lifestyle.

The Role of GnRH, Norepinephrine, and Beta Endorphin

The hypothalamus is the thermoregulation center and great regulator of the HPO axis. Aging and erratic hormone-level fluctuations within this system affect GnRH and cause it to lose its ability to keep a consistent pulse. Once the GnRH pulse generator becomes interrupted, the HPO axis has even greater difficulty maintaining balance during menopausal transition:

> Alterations of the GnRH pulse generator and regulatory (both excitatory and inhibitory) neuropeptides might contribute to the compromise or complete absence of the mid-cycle LH surge, also consistent with a reduction in the sensitivity of the hypothalamus and pituitary to positive feedback by estrogen. (North American Menopause Society 2014, p.9)

The pulse gradually becomes slower and then releases more GnRH per pulse. This is a yin and yang imbalance. Erratic GnRH pulse fluctuations make it difficult for the hypothalamus to maintain normal control of body thermoregulation. This is like trying to maintain a consistent car speed in traffic with frequent speeding up and slowing down.

Norepinephrine plays an important role in thermoregulation. Norepinephrine functions in the brain and body as a hormone and as the main neurotransmitter used by the sympathetic nervous system.

Norepinephrine release is lowest during sleep (yin) and rises during wakefulness (yang).

High levels of norepinephrine happen during situations of stress, fear, or danger. In this way, stress directly affects the HPO axis and sympathetic nervous system. High levels of norepinephrine affect alertness, memory and attention, restlessness and anxiety, heart rate, blood pressure, and blood flow.

Norepinephrine levels have a direct effect on thermoregulation. α2 adrenergic antagonists elevate brain norepinephrine and trigger hot flashes, while α2 agonists ameliorate hot flashes.

> Elevated central sympathetic activation, mediated through α2-adr-energic receptors, is one factor responsible for narrowing of the thermoneutral zone… Norepinephrine (NE) plays an important role in thermoregulation acting, in part, through α2-adrenergic receptors. (Freedman 2014)

Norepinephrine and sympathetic-nervous-system excitation have a direct link to thermoregulation problems and are direct causes of hot flashes. The warranted treatment is to decrease sympathetic-nervous-system excitation by returning to a parasympathetic state. This is done in Chinese medicine by sedating excessive yang qi and calming the spirit.

Elevated brain norepinephrine and estrogen withdrawal are prime components of hot flash etiology (Freedman 2014). Norepinephrine acts like yang qi, and estrogen acts like yin qi. Together, norepinephrine and estrogen play a central role in neuroregulation or balancing the yin and yang activity of the brain.

Beta endorphin or β-endorphin is an endogenous opioid neuropeptide that functions in the central nervous system to regulate stress and maintain homeostasis. Decreased β-endorphin levels are linked to a decrease in estrogen concentrations. Reductions in β-endorphin levels "affect the thermoregulatory center in the hypothalamus and allow increases in gonadotropin-releasing hormone pulse rates and amplitude" (Avis and Coeytaux 2010, p.228) and "increase the release of serotonin and norepinephrine, and this may in turn cause a drop in the set point in the thermoregulatory center in the hypothalamus and elicit inappropriate heat loss" (Borud *et al.* 2009, p.491).

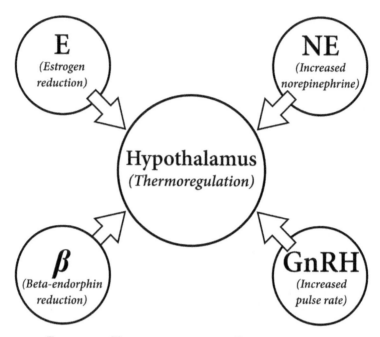

FIGURE 4.2: THERMOREGULATION—PATHOMECHANISMS

The reduction of estrogen concentrations during menopausal transition has a decreasing effect on β-endorphin levels, which increases GnRH pulse rates and norepinephrine levels, narrowing the thermoneutral zone within the hypothalamus.

Acupuncture has a positive effect on thermoregulation with its stimulating effect on β-endorphin and estrogen, regulatory effect on GnRH, and sedative effect on norepinephrine. Supporting proper brain neuroregulation, quality blood supplementation to the brain, and blood flow within the brain all help ameliorate the hot-flash environment.

Reproductive Aging

Insight into the menstrual cycle and its mechanisms provides a better understanding of the natural reproductive aging process. The reproductive aging process is a natural occurrence that takes place in all women. The age when this starts varies and the process may be faster or slower depending on the individual. The menstrual cycle becomes irregular for most women by the mid to late forties and eventually stops in their early fifties.

Stages of Reproductive Aging Workshop +10 Staging System (STRAW +10)

STRAW provides a comprehensive basis for assessing and understanding reproductive aging in women (Harlow *et al.* 2012). It is broken into ten stages within three main categories: reproductive years, menopausal transition, and post-menopause. By taking a closer look at each step in the ten stages and highlighting the changing mechanisms, it provides useful information and an understanding of the causes and the formation of hot flashes.

The reproductive years are divided into three stages: early (−5), peak (−4), and late (−3b and −3a) stages. The early and peak stages are normal reproductive years of a woman's life. The hormones are balanced, there's an ample supply of follicles, and the menstrual cycle is for the most part regular. Subtle changes start to appear with the hormones and the menstrual cycle during the late reproductive stages. The menstrual cycle begins to show changes in length and flow, measurable anti-mullerian hormone and antral follicle count levels begin to decline, and inhibin B levels drop, causing the FSH levels to rise and become variable.

In Chinese medicine, we can understand these changes as the decrease in estrogen from the ovary (yin), with a subsequent decline in inhibin B, causing FSH secretion from the pituitary gland to rise (yang); thus creating a yin deficiency yang excess state based on Western medicine. This is the foundation for hot flashes and menopause symptoms.

The menopausal transition years are divided into two stages: early (−2) and late (−1) stages. This time period is considered "perimenopause." The menstrual cycle becomes increasingly irregular and is accompanied by increased hormone-secretion variability. The central nervous system and ovarian follicular atresia are considered the source of these changes. These changes increase yang hyperactivity and the depletion of yin.

The length of the cycle is the most noticeable symptom during menopausal transition. This is due to the increased variable levels of estrogen and FSH; the two hormones are trying to balance the menstrual cycle. The estrogen levels continue to decline, so the FSH is trying to overcompensate by overstimulating the ovary to produce a mature follicle, creating violent pushing and pulling on the system. This is what causes the cycle to become shorter, longer, and erratic.

In the early stage, the cycle becomes persistently irregular, with the length being noticeably (seven or more days) longer or shorter for ten or more cycles. A woman enters the late stage once the cycle begins to skip periods, which is called amenorrhea, especially if two or more periods in a row are skipped. The cause is low estrogen and progesterone and elevated FSH and LH imbalance. The average length of menopausal transition is one to three years.

Post-menopause years are divided into two stages: early (+1a, +1b, +1c) and late (+2) stages. The early stage (+1a) is marked as the transition from menopausal transition late stage to post-menopause, which is marked by the FMP. This is the cumulative effect of the hormones on the endometrium. The FMP is calculated amenorrhea, or no periods, for a duration of 12 months. +1b and +1c mark the next two to six years post-FMP. It is the early stages of post-menopause when the estrogen and FSH become stabilized and when hot flashes and other VMS commonly start. The late (+2) stage marks the rest of a woman's life.

Western-Medicine Treatment Approaches

It is not the intention of this book to explain and decipher Western medical treatments. An overview is more than adequate to gain an understanding about the different therapies and treatment strategies, including contraceptives, HT, and nonpharmacological treatments. The objective is to highlight possible shortcomings of the Western system, and the risks and benefits, and hopefully show reasons to utilize acupuncture and Chinese herbal medicine as alternatives.

A Note on Pharmaceuticals

Pharmaceuticals are chemicals and are significantly more potent than herbal medicine. They produce strong reactions in the body. Some carry great efficacy and are vital for treatment, while others offer little advantage for the patient.

Many drug-induced actions are not achievable with normal herbal medicines and healthy lifestyle changes. These strong reactions can be accompanied by negative side effects that are unresponsive to acupuncture and Chinese herbal medicine. It is extremely difficult, morally, legally, and ethically as a doctor of acupuncture and Chinese herbal medicine, to comment on or make suggestions to patients regarding Western drugs.

The good news is that we can utilize acupuncture and herbal formulas in conjunction with pharmaceuticals without serious interactions. It is up to the practitioner to know and understand where there may be potential contraindications.

Contraceptives

Contraceptives are mainly used during the reproductive years to prevent pregnancy. They are also prescribed during menopausal transition to control heavy and irregular menstrual bleeding.

The benefits to using contraceptives during menopausal transition are regulating irregular uterine bleeding, dysmenorrhea, reducing VMS including hot flashes, decreasing the risk of ovarian, breast, and endometrial cancer, and maintaining bone density.

Common side effects from contraceptive use include headaches, genital irritation, fatigue, mood changes, changes in the period, bloating, withdrawal bleeding and spotting, cramping, breast tenderness, difficulty returning to fertility, nausea, libido issues, depression, weight gain, and nervousness.

To avoid potential risks, contraindications for contraceptive use include hypertension, diabetes, stroke, obesity, venous thromboembolism, hormone-dependent cancers, abnormal uterine bleeding, smoking, and heart disease.

HT

HT is currently considered the most effective treatment of hot flashes. There are two categories of HT: estrogen therapy (ET) and estrogen-progestogen therapy (EPT). ET is used for women who have gone through a hysterectomy. EPT has the addition of progestogen to reduce the risk of endometrial adenocarcinoma in women with an intact uterus. "Use of HT after menopause is considered therapeutic for menopausal symptoms, not replacement for a deficiency state" (North American Menopause Society 2014, p.263).

ET reestablishes the function of estrogen in the body, including growth in the reproductive area, and acts on the HPO axis. It is used for moderate to severe VMS, vaginal dryness, vulvovaginal atrophy, painful intercourse, urinary urgency, dysuria, and osteoporosis.

ET is another option to treat VMS and is commonly used to target the uterus to convert estrogen to reduce the risk of endometrial cancers.

EPT is the current clinical standard treatment for VMS. The goal is to provide uterine protection, maintain estrogen benefits for the body, and minimize adverse events, particularly uterine bleeding. It should not be relied on to reduce cardiovascular disease or risk of breast cancer.

There are many contraindications for the use of EPT, including a history of breast or endometrial cancer, abnormal genital bleeding, estrogen-dependent neoplasia, deep vein thrombosis, pulmonary embolism, arterial thromboembolic disease, liver dysfunction, pregnancy, and hypersensitivity to ET or EPT.

The Women's Health Initiative

The Women's Health Initiative (WHI) conducted the largest clinical trials on the use and effects of HT in the early 1990s. The trials were discontinued once results started showing that HT posed many potentially serious health risks.

HT has a complex pattern of risks and benefits. The results for EPT were an increased risk for breast cancer, stroke, heart attack, and blood clots. The results for ET were an increased risk for stroke and venous thrombosis. Both therapies carried a higher risk of cognitive impairment and dementia.

There are many types, combinations, and routes of administration for HT. The collected scientific research surrounding HT is widely variable. Even though HT carries many potential and unknown health risks, it is still popular and widely prescribed to treat VMS.

Women must evaluate and weigh the benefits and risks of HT. For a woman with typical VMS, treatment is appropriate and can be relatively straightforward, with a short course of HT usually being sufficient. Treatment should be halted or discontinued if symptoms occur that pose a health risk.

HT can be very effective for relieving hot flashes: "Estrogen plus progestogen therapy relieves hot flash intensity by approximately 90%" (Borud *et al.* 2009, p.484; Maclennan *et al.* 2004). It can be fast and more effective than acupuncture and Chinese herbal medicine. It does, though, carry serious risks, especially in long-term treatment, including coronary heart disease, breast cancer, stroke, and blood clots (Rossouw *et al.* 2002). This is the main reason to consider acupuncture and Chinese herbal medicine as the primary treatment method.

My clinical experience suggests there is less need for HT and greater need for practitioners to guide patients in concrete lifestyle changes. Acupuncture and Chinese herbal medicine, and many natural and proactive therapies such as meditation, yoga, exercise, stress reduction, and relaxation techniques, can help reestablish brain activity and balance the neuro-endocrine system.

Bioidentical Hormone Therapy (BHT)

"Bioidentical hormones" means that all hormones used are "chemically identical" to those made in the human body. BHT is also considered a "specialized and individualized" HT, tailored specifically for each patient.

Many experts consider BHT safe and natural. The United States Food and Drug Administration (FDA) claims that the chemical compounds are exactly the same as HT and pose a greater public risk because they are unregulated (Pinkerton 2012).

BHT became widely popular after the WHI findings. BHT is

frequently used and prescribed in many nonconventional Western medical clinics. BHT products carry the same risks as regular HT products.

Selective Estrogen-Receptor Modulators (SERMs)

SERMs are estrogen-like compounds that act as estrogen agonists or antagonists, depending on the SERM and targeted tissue. They are used primarily to target, prevent, and treat several diseases, including breast cancer, osteoporosis, dyspareunia, and VMS. SERMs are less commonly used in the treatment of hot flashes and carry increased risks of blood clots, stroke, and endometrial cancer.

SSRIs and SNRIs

SSRIs and SNRIs are largely used to treat depression and anxiety disorders. They work by increasing serotonin or norepinephrine levels, the neurotransmitters in the brain involved in happiness and mood. Over the past two decades, they have increasingly been used to treat moderate to severe VMS with modest yet temporary improvements (Joffe *et al.* 2013; Shams *et al.* 2014). It should be noted that there is little quality research regarding safety and adverse effects with long-term use of SSRIs and SNRIs.

Predisposed Menopause and Artificial Menopause

Some women are naturally more predisposed to hot flashes than other women, whether they are genetic (pre-heaven qi) or due to lifestyle choices (post-heaven qi). Cases of premature menopause generally fall into this category. This goes along with the saying "It runs in the family." This phrase is only partly true and is inconclusive.

A woman can be predisposed based on family genetics, but the deciding factor is often her lifestyle habits over the course of her life. The reason many women experience similar menopausal-transition symptoms is because of their upbringing and similar lifestyle habits.

Hot flashes can also be created and induced by medical interventions that cause artificial menopause.

A partial hysterectomy is the removal of the uterus only. A total hysterectomy is the removal of the uterus and cervix. They usually do not induce hot flashes. When the ovaries are still intact, they are able to release estrogen and maintain the HPO axis. In Chinese medicine, the underlying pattern that created the need for the hysterectomy is still there and will likely be the cause of increased perimenopausal symptoms and an earlier-than-normal onset of menopausal transition.

A total hysterectomy and bilateral salpingo-oophorectomy is the removal of the uterus, cervix, ovaries, and fallopian tubes. With the removal of the ovaries, the blood serum estrogen levels dramatically decline, creating an instant shift in the HPO axis. Menopausal transition instantaneously starts after this procedure, skipping the early stages. The menstrual cycle stops and VMS, including hot flashes, frequently begin immediately and sometimes with great intensity. One study suggests a rise in serum FSH and hot flashes in total-hysterectomy women, creating a link to FSH levels and hot flashes (Halmesmäki et al. 2004). In Chinese medicine, FSH is yang oriented and rising yang qi can overstimulate the brain and harass the heart qi.

It is necessary to start acupuncture treatments directly following a total hysterectomy and bilateral salpingo-oophorectomy in order to control hot-flash severity. The longer a patient waits before receiving acupuncture treatment, the longer the hot-flash environment has to become established, and it becomes increasingly difficult to regain control of thermoregulation. It is worth noting here that depending on the age and timing of a patient's total hysterectomy and bilateral salpingo-oophorectomy, it is likely for them to experience a second spike in VMS around normal menopausal transition age.

Chemotherapy and Radiation Treatments

Chemotherapy and radiation treatment for cancer can generate menopausal-transition signs and symptoms, such as hot flashes and cessation of periods, during the course of treatment. Chemotherapy and radiation consume and damage the yuan qi and introduce high levels of heat toxins to the body, which creates a heat repletion and stagnation hot-flash environment.

Hot flashes are one of the most common and distressing symptoms experienced by up to 73% of breast cancer survivors after cancer treatment... Some cancer treatments, such as surgery, chemotherapy, and antiestrogen therapies, disrupt estrogen synthesis and activity, which can result in severe hot flashes. (Romero *et al.* 2020, p.913)

Conclusion

Effectively treating hot flashes and regaining control of the thermoneutral zone consists of the following factors.

- Balancing the sympathetic and parasympathetic nervous system to open the thermoneutral zone.

- Soothing the hypothalamus to relax its restraint on thermoregulation.

- Assisting the hypothalamus and pituitary gland in overcoming their dependence on estrogen while stimulating circulating β-endorphin and estrogen levels.

- Regulating and sedating chaotic neurotransmitter communication within the brain.

Treating dysregulation requires the balancing of yin and yang. Treating deficiency requires supplementation of qi, blood, yin, yang, and essence. Treating stagnation requires the moving of qi and blood. Each woman has a unique combination of these factors, and effective treatment requires the creation of individualized acupuncture, herbal medicine, and lifestyle modification plans.

• Chapter 5 •

Hot Flashes—Chinese-Medicine Diagnosis

Introduction

A theory is just that—speculation. It is merely an idea until it is brought into a real-life situation. Chinese medicine is a vast universe, rich in theory. It would require many lifetimes of study to master it all. To be a successful Chinese medical doctor, acupuncturist, and herbal medicine practitioner, it is necessary not only to read and comprehend the history and theory, but also to test it by putting it to use.

To try and fail over and over is part of practicing medicine. Treating and helping people is a gift. Not a gift of talent but one of privilege. It is up to the practitioner to bring their knowledge of Chinese-medicine theory out of the books and into the clinic to bring it to life. Only by applying their knowledge can a practitioner become a healer. The following passage from the *Neijing Lingshu* beautifully illustrates this concept:

> Those who are able to distinguish between yin and yang associations of the twelve conduits, they know why/where a disease emerges. Those who look for the locations of conditions of depletion and repletion, they are able to recognize whether an illness is located above or below. Those who know the qi paths of the six short-term repositories, they know how to untie knots, tie ends, and ensure security at the gateways. Those who know how a condition of depletion and repletion is associated with hardness and softness, they know where to supplement and

where to drain. Those who know about tips and root [of diseases] in the six conduits, they are not confused by anything on earth. *Neijing Lingshu*, Chapter 52 (Unschuld 2016a, p.502)

Diagnosing and treating menopausal-transition patients is both frustrating and enjoyable, easy and difficult. Chinese-medicine theory provides a solid foundation for the practitioner to stand upon to be able to understand the condition of each individual patient. But using theory and understanding to develop a diagnosis produces something much more valuable, the necessary compass for the practitioner to navigate through the treatment of the patient. Without this guidance, the practitioner's healing ability will plateau.

The diagnosis information that follows is not a simple recipe—it is a map for the clinician. It is up to the clinician to decide which road to take.

Effective Hot-Flash Diagnosis

The clinician has two goals: correctly diagnosing the hot-flash environment and administering successful treatment to quell the hot flash. Effective diagnosis depends on the clinician investigating several factors of the patient's overall health history and current medical condition.

A thorough clinical hot-flash diagnosis must consider:

- congenital factors, such as genetics and family history

- past medical history and factors, such as childhood diseases, nutrition, and chemical and environmental exposures

- past and present lifestyle factors, such as work and rest, diet and exercise, stress and emotional stability, medications, and overall health

- past and current gynecological medical history

- a full internal medical history.

Discussing medical and lifestyle history provides insight and a clearer understanding of each patient's imbalance and hot-flash environment for an accurate diagnosis.

As we will see, every patient will have their own unique excesses and deficiencies, stagnation, and imbalances of yin and yang. Although many are similar, no two patients are exactly the same. A specific and individualized diagnosis allows the practitioner to administer a personalized acupuncture prescription and herbal formula.

Diagnosing the hot-flash patient is an artful journey of discovery to a clear understanding of the patient's hot-flash environment. We have discussed in depth the many physiological patterns contributing to the hot flash. We can now combine this knowledge with our diagnostic tools to correctly hone in on the nature and cause.

The Congenital and Acquired Constitutions

Our constitution is the combined physical, mental, and spiritual foundation of our body. Our overall health is an outward expression and manifestation of our constitution. Taking care of one's health is taking care of one's constitution.

Some of our constitution is largely set in stone at the genetic level, while we have the direct ability to adapt, affect, and change other aspects of our constitution. Sometimes this can happen quickly over a few split seconds, while sometimes it requires gradual change over months or years. Improving and maintaining our health is a privilege and should be met with grace. Some changes happen easily, while others are only achieved with difficulty.

Seeing and knowing the patient's overall constitution allows the practitioner to understand the patient's hot-flash environment. It allows for a correct diagnosis of the pattern, and the practitioner will have strong indications of how well the patient will respond even before starting treatment.

Pre-Heaven or Earlier Heaven Constitution

The pre-heaven (congenital) constitution is formed before we are born and is related to the kidney. It is made from the combined essence of our mother and father. It is unique in the sense that the essence from each parent is a direct manifestation of their qi at the moment of our conception. Their essence is a combination of their pre-heaven and post-heaven qi.

The quality of our qi has the capability to positively and adversely affect our essence. It is especially important to take care of one's post-heaven qi before conceiving a child. This is so the essence being passed on to one's child is as good as it can be for "optimal genetic essence."

The pre-heaven constitution derives from genetics and family history. Other factors can influence it. Things such as trauma during delivery, a premature birth, or in-utero issues such as nutritional deficiencies, impairments, or exposure to harmful substances can affect the overall pre-heaven constitution.

It is important to ask questions about these potential problems in the clinic. Pre-heaven constitution deficiencies are difficult to repair, and problems due to these deficiencies can be just as difficult to treat. If the patient has healthy lifestyle habits, generates optimal qi, and has a strong post-heaven constitution, this can be redirected back into the mingmen and, over time, repair the pre-heaven essence.

Post-Heaven or Later Heaven Constitution

The post-heaven (acquired) constitution comprises our physical, mental, and spiritual strengths and weaknesses and marks our overall health. It is related to the lung and spleen. The overall strength of our pre-heaven constitution has a direct influence on the performance of our post-heaven constitution.

For example, if someone has a weak pre-heaven qi, it is natural for them to begin life with a weakened post-heaven qi state. The post-heaven constitution is generated once we are born. After that, our overall lifestyle habits are in charge of maintaining our constitution.

The post-heaven constitution is generally what we see and think about when we have a health problem. It is what we diagnose and treat in the clinical setting.

Past and present medical problems will have an influence on the post-heaven constitution. Factors such as a history of chronic or severe illnesses, high fevers, infectious diseases, pathogenic factors, physical or emotional trauma, accidents, loss of blood, surgeries, allergies, and exposure to environmental and chemical toxins can all affect the post-heaven constitution. This is why it is essential to carefully examine the patient's medical history.

The strengths and weaknesses of the two constitutions blend together, and the constitution is supported by the continual efforts of the lung-spleen-kidney axis. This is why both pre-heaven and post-heaven constitution issues can be resolved or damaged by lifestyle habits.

The Five Zang—Lifestyle Habits

Our lifestyle habits have a direct effect on our overall health constitution. Good health is the result of taking good care of ourselves.

Healthy lifestyle habits are a necessity for an optimal menopausal transition. Positive lifestyle changes are the ideal medical interventions. They pose no health risks. They can prevent hot flashes or reduce severity, frequency, and duration. Healthy habits can balance brain neuroregulation by building healthy and quality qi and blood.

Lifestyle habits fall in conjunction with the five zang organs in Chinese medicine. Exercise, routine activity, and breath work affect the lung. Relaxation techniques, stress reduction, and meditation affect the liver. A healthy, clean diet and hydration affect the spleen. Balanced work and rest habits, and adequate rest, affect the kidney. Finding a sense of joy and purpose in life affects the heart. All are proven measures for supporting good health.

Menopausal transition is directly affected by the overall strength of the congenital and acquired qi, and women enter into menopausal transition with either a strong or weakened constitution. Women who enter menopausal transition with an established healthy constitution and habits, or who improve and sustain their health and well-being with positive lifestyle habits, generally go through the transition with fewer difficulties.

The Lung: Activity and Breath

A healthy and active lifestyle is not all about going to the health club and participating in cardio activities and lifting weights. This works for some people but not for all. It is more about quality activity that helps regulate the breath and circulates the qi and blood. Walking, hiking, yoga, gardening, and other low-impact activities that are healthy and enjoyable produce positive effects with less wear and tear on the body over the long term.

When the qi connection between the lung and the kidney is established, the qi will flow without hesitation, the zangfu organs will generate an abundance of qi and blood, and the spirit will be calm. You should feel happier and healthier after partaking in exercise and activity that you enjoy.

The Spleen: Diet and Nutrition

Healthy digestion generates blood and nutrition for the body. Food and water serve as the primary source and foundation for our qi and blood. Healthy dietary choices provide our body with quality nutrition.

Our dietary choices and habits will have both short-term and long-term effects on our overall health and constitution. Choices consist primarily of what we eat, while habits are about how often and how much we eat.

When we eat a diet rich in nutrients and devoid of junk and maintain regular eating habits, without overeating or skipping meals, we can support our spleen in generating quality qi and blood. You should feel energized and healthier when your dietary lifestyle is in rhythm.

The Kidney: Work and Rest

A healthy balance of work and rest throughout the day allows proper regeneration and distribution of the kidney essence. Working long hours without breaks, not taking vacations, or depriving ourselves of adequate sleep slowly consumes the kidney essence over time.

Both physical and mental overwork directly and indirectly weaken the kidney, whether it's sitting behind a desk and computer all day or actively participating in long hours of physical labor. The kidney essence and vital qi will be permanently damaged when people do not take the necessary breaks throughout the day and maintain quality rest and sleep.

Maintaining physical and mental rest through the days, weeks, months, and years allows the kidney to recharge and for the essence and vital qi to rebuild. When the kidney has adequate time to build essence, they can in turn support the rest of the zangfu organs.

The Liver: Stress and Emotions

We all require positive ways to help maintain emotional stability and balance daily stresses. It is easy for some while challenging for others. Relaxing techniques such as exercise, acupuncture, massage, change in surroundings, meditation, talking, solitude, rest, or participating in a mindful activity can all produce positive health effects.

When we are able to deal with short-term and long-term stress and emotional imbalances in a positive way, our liver will be able to regulate qi and balance yin and yang throughout the body. Uninhibited qi flow throughout the body is paramount to health. This allows the zangfu organ system to perform its duties without hesitation and creates an environment for a peaceful spirit.

The Heart: Joy and Purpose

Finding and possessing a sense of purpose in life opens the heart and spirit; there is no greater feeling in life. We are at peace when our heart is filled with joy and happiness.

When the heart is filled with joy, it relaxes and allows the qi and blood to circulate throughout the body. When the qi and blood can move without issue, the zangfu organs will generate an abundance of qi and blood, and the spirit will be calm. To reach this state is the purpose of our existence.

Diagnosing Hot-Flash Patterns
Relative and True Yin Deficiency

There are two types of yin deficiency: both relative and true yin deficiency can create a hot-flash environment. Relative yin is like the water within a well. True yin is like the water in the aquifer seated deep beneath the well.

Relative yin deficiency can appear in almost every zangfu organ and is not bound to the aging process. Relative yin deficiency can be seen in any patient. It is termed "relative" yin deficiency because it can happen at any age and comes and goes as the result of many lifestyle and environmental factors and is often easily remedied. As the yin (water) declines, the yang (fire) increases. If left unabated, over time this yin deficient heat slowly dries out the organs and tissues.

Relative yin deficiency is the result of long-standing lifestyle habits and environmental factors. For example, many hot-flash patients present in the clinic with stomach yin deficiency. This pattern is due to irregular dietary and eating habits including overeating, undereating, skipping meals, dehydration, and consuming foods and beverages that are drying in nature such as coffee and tea, processed foods, and alcohol. The stomach sits below the heart, and when the heat smolders in the stomach, it rises and agitates the heart fire.

Herein lies the traditional menopausal-transition pattern described throughout contemporary Chinese medicine.

Relative yin deficiency heat or fire may be mild or particularly intense in nature depending on the circumstance. It makes hot flashes stronger by amplifying the true underlying pattern. Diagnosing and targeting relative yin deficiency based on the affected individual zangfu organs is easy, and it responds well to acupuncture and herbal medicine.

True yin deficiency is the decline of the original yin of the kidney. This original yin is the foundation and source of yin for the rest of the body.

Some people are born with a pre-heaven true yin deficiency. This is a result of a genetic, in-utero, or birthing issue. It is essential to ask patients the right questions to determine if there were any issues in these areas, specifically in-utero or birthing trauma, premature birth, nutritional deficiencies from the mother, or other family traits that would have led to the taxation of original yin.

Post-heaven true yin deficiency can happen from the aging process, a serious or long-standing consumptive illness, extreme taxation to the body, or a traumatic event.

Severe illness, long-standing illness, severe taxation to the body, or a physical or psychological traumatic event that consumes large amounts of the vital original yin can result in true yin deficiency. It is important to question patients about infections, high fevers, severe illnesses, traumas, loss of blood, surgeries, extreme physical activities, drug use, and physical and emotional traumas to determine if their medical history suggests possible absolute yin deficiency.

Tidal heat effusion due to true yin deficiency is more severe and difficult to treat than relative yin deficiency. If the true yin deficiency is damaged at a young age or is due to a pre-heaven issue, these patients will experience hot-flash symptoms at a much earlier age and can present with severe hot flashes during perimenopause and menopausal transition. If the true yin is damaged later in life, possibly by severe illness or cancer treatments, patients will experience hot flashes well into post-menopause. These patients may require treatments over a longer course of time and with gentler treatment approaches to quell the hot flashes.

The original yin and yang naturally decline over time because of the aging process. This is quite apparent in the elderly population. This decline due to aging is not, however, usually a factor in menopausal transition, which occurs at an age when many patients' original yin is still intact. In fact, it is more common to see the natural effects of true yin deficiency begin to start when the patient reaches post-menopause or beyond. The use of yin tonics doesn't necessarily work for treating hot flashes during menopausal transition because they are being used too early in the aging process.

Yang Exuberance

There are two types of yang exuberance that can create or add to the hot-flash environment: yin deficiency yang rising patterns and excessive yang qi patterns. Yang exuberance patterns, in general, co-incide with yin deficiency patterns.

Yang exuberance has the natural tendency to ascend. This ascension has the potential to harass the upper portions of the body, including the head, brain, sensory organs, and heart. It has the potential to bring heat upwards with it. Deficiency of yin generates heat, and the ascending yang moves this heat upwards and fuels the heart fire.

This describes the yin deficiency yang rising hot-flash pattern. This is the most common hot-flash environment scenario.

Excessive yang qi patterns are of a different nature, as they can be a pattern of excess and are not necessarily tied to a deficiency of yin state. The primary source of this hyperactive yang is the liver. It becomes exuberant from liver qi stagnation or fire, which may include liver yin or blood deficiency and heat repletion or damp-phlegm complications. Excessive yang qi can also develop from excess and stagnation in the fu organs.

Lifestyle habits are the most common source of qi stagnation. Qi stagnation generates fire. This creates a vicious cycle: qi stagnation and fire stir yang qi, which in turn further influences and agitates emotions and lifestyle habits. It can be a difficult cycle to break if the patient is unaware of how their choices and behaviors control it.

Hot flashes due to excessive yang qi patterns are more severe than yin deficiency yang rising patterns, because it is an excess pattern. Excess patterns often do respond well and quickly to treatments. It is worth noting, though, that these hot-flash patients may require routine treatments, as the hot flashes will return if certain lifestyle changes are not made to break the cycle.

Yang excess symptoms are more prominent in perimenopause patients. Over time, excessive yang qi patterns will consume yin, creating an excess deficiency situation. Hot flashes will be more severe in nature and more resistant to treatments when yang qi is excessive and the yin deficiency becomes more pronounced.

Yang Deficiency

Yang deficiency is the unseen culprit of many hot-flash scenarios. Yang deficiency is insidious because it mimics yin deficient yang exuberance cases. The fire smolders within water because yang cannot engender yin. Patients in this category are yang deficient in nature but present with yin excess and fire. It can easily be misdiagnosed as a damp-heat or stirring of ministerial fire pattern.

Yang deficiency takes a long time to develop for the menopausal-transition patient. There are two causes: overwork and poor lifestyle habits.

Patients with yang deficiency due to overwork commonly present with the classical qi or yang deficiency pattern and symptoms. It is sometimes surprising when these patients mention they are experiencing hot flashes. Patients in this category enjoy activity, as it makes them feel better, and also benefit from rest.

Patients with yang deficiency due to poor lifestyle habits do not present with a qi or yang deficiency pattern. This is because their deficiency state, over time, has generated a stagnative, excessive, and fire-enhanced environment. These patients generally live a sedentary lifestyle and are resistant to activity, while most work long hours and have less time to practice a healthy lifestyle. Once they make the time and make their health a priority, they may be able to make the connection between more activity and a healthier lifestyle, and feeling better.

Hot flashes due to yang deficiency respond poorly when treatments target heat symptoms. Even though the patient may be presenting with heat and excess symptoms, it is necessary to administer yang engendering therapies to quell the hot flashes. Simple acupuncture techniques, herbal formulas, and positive lifestyle changes provide effective relief for these patients.

Qi and Blood Deficiency

Qi and blood deficiency is a common occurrence. It plays a large underlying role in the hot-flash environment. Living in our modern society has the tendency to consume qi and blood at an accelerated pace. That is why it is important to maintain a balance of activity, rest, healthy dietary choices, and stress management, and strive for a sense of joy, purpose, and accomplishment. These practices help women regenerate a healthy supply of qi and blood following its loss from the monthly period.

Qi and blood deficiency can generate hot flashes in a number of ways. Healthy qi has the ability to control and maintain the balance of yin and yang. Balance diminishes when qi becomes weak, resulting in bursts of yang qi, especially when yang is exuberant. A perfect example is a qi deficient patient with increased morning hot flashes. Tonifying qi will abate the hot flashes.

Blood comprises yin and yang components. Blood deficiency will offset the internal yin and yang equilibrium and generate hot flashes in two ways. First, blood has a cooling function, being yin in nature. If blood becomes deficient, much like yin deficiency, its yin ability to nourish and cool the tissues will diminish, while its yang tendency to heat up the tissues will increase. This is a deficiency of yin within yin. Second, yang resides within the blood (yang within yin) and is warming in nature. When yang qi within the blood is exuberant, due to original yang qi exuberance or blood deficiency, it will increase in temperature and speed up circulation. This will heat up the surface and upper portions of the body and fuel the heart fire. This is an excess of yang within yin. Hot flashes of this nature will be stronger than those of yin within yin.

Hot flashes due to qi and blood deficiency are most often mild in nature and respond favorably to acupuncture and herbal medicine. In fact, many women will resolve their hot flashes by simply addressing lifestyle habits that nourish qi and blood.

Stagnation

Stagnations encompass a large group of patterns primarily consisting of irregular flow of qi: qi stagnation, blood stasis, damp-phlegm accumulation, cold, heat, or fire. Stagnations have the tendency to combine with one another to create further complexities. Stagnations are the result of excess or deficiency dysfunction within the yin and yang, qi and blood, channel system, or the zangfu organs.

Stagnation is the primary cause of perimenopausal hot flashes and complicates menopausal-transition hot flashes. Lifestyle choices are often the main source of stagnations, including lack of activity, poor dietary choices, dehydration, high stress and emotional imbalances, and lack of rest. They do respond quite well to acupuncture, but oftentimes return if proper lifestyle adjustments are not made.

Stagnations can directly create hot flashes and indirectly enhance the hot-flash environment. When qi cannot flow freely, over time, its yang energy builds and generates heat. At a certain point, like a pressure cooker, the heat is released. This rush of heat ascends upwards and outwards as a direct form of a hot flash.

Stagnations indirectly enhance existing hot flashes and further complicate any previous underlying situations. When qi cannot move freely, it loses its ability to control the balance of yin and yang, promote circulation of blood and body fluids, and maintain proper stability and communication between the internal zangfu organs.

Finally, chronic and severe cases of stagnation will involve phlegm and fire. This situation will harass the heart and cause spirit disorders. This situation can produce stubborn, frequent, and intractable hot flashes.

Unfortunately, many of the smaller, lesser, or minor stagnations in the body are undetectable to the practitioner and perhaps the patient is blind to them as well. These minor stagnations due to habitual lifestyle skew the qi dynamic network. It is apparent in the breath, sleep patterns, spirit, digestion, and physical and mental aspects. Minor stagnations are routine and part of life. If and once the patient is able to witness and tap into the problem, they are able to remedy it.

Axis, Trajectories, and Triads

The axis, trajectories, and triads are six specific groups comprised of three zang organs. Each group comes together based on distinctive yin and yang connections, qi and blood circulation and generation, and excess and deficiency physiological relationships. Together, their combined efforts generate and move qi and blood throughout the body.

The axis, trajectories, and triads function to systematically diagnose certain aspects of the hot-flash environment. Utilizing them in conjunction with one another helps improve the diagnosis process. It serves to compartmentalize problematic areas and is a way to stay consistent with diagnosis and treatments.

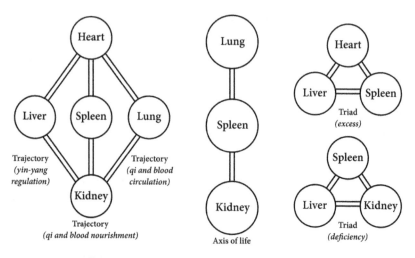

FIGURE 5.1: AXIS, TRAJECTORIES, AND TRIADS

The Lung-Spleen-Kidney Axis

The first group is the lung-spleen-kidney axis and what I call the "axis of life." These are the three primary organs in charge of generating yuan (source) qi. Based on breath, nutrition, and activity, when these three organs are working optimally and in harmony, the yuan qi they create is the foundational qi that in turn supports the qi and blood, yin and yang, and essence throughout the entire body.

The lung, spleen, and kidney need continuous support and are prone to qi and blood deficiency and deficiency-influenced stagnations. It is necessary to support these three organs if the patient shows general signs of fatigue and other qi and blood deficiency signs. Proper activity, diet, and rest habits tailored for the individual are paramount to keep these organs healthy.

The Three Trajectories

The second set of groups is what I call trajectories. The three trajectories are three distinct zang organ pathways linking the kidney to the heart. The clinician needs to give close attention to these two primary organs when diagnosing and treating hot flashes.

The three trajectories are used to diagnose: yin and yang balance; qi and blood nourishment; qi and blood circulation.

THE KIDNEY-LIVER-HEART TRAJECTORY
The kidney-liver-heart trajectory serves as the yin and yang equalizer between the chest and mingmen. The heart and kidney have a continual yin and yang (water and fire) exchange, but are susceptible to imbalance during menopausal transition. It is within this trajectory that the water-fire is kept in balance. The liver is in the center of the two and serves to regulate the relative excess and deficiency of yin and yang.

Mental and emotional excitement and exhaustion play a central role in this trajectory. The patient's sleep patterns and emotional state will help the clinician decide if sedation or tonification is warranted to maintain yin and yang balance.

THE KIDNEY-SPLEEN-HEART TRAJECTORY
The kidney-spleen-heart trajectory serves to directly supply adequate qi and blood nourishment from the kidney to the heart via the spleen. The yang qi fire within the mingmen helps the kidney essence ascend to combine with the refined qi of the spleen to generate qi and blood. This fresh qi and blood is then pushed further upwards to the heart. It is within this trajectory that the heart is properly and abundantly nourished. The spleen and kidney are under continual pressure to replenish qi and blood lost due to the menstrual cycle. They are prone to deficiencies. These three organs help nourish and calm the spirit.

THE KIDNEY-LUNG-HEART TRAJECTORY
The kidney-lung-heart trajectory functions to maintain healthy qi and blood circulation to and from the heart and out to the rest of the body via the channel system. This is based on two factors. First, the lung and heart govern qi and blood and its circulation. Second, the lung and kidney respiration propels the qi and blood through the vessels. It is within this trajectory that the zangfu organs and the rest of the body can function optimally.

The zangfu organs and channel system rely on the proper qi and blood circulation. Circulation is susceptible to deficiency and stagnation, which can create problems with the menstrual cycle and menopausal transition.

The kidney-spleen-heart trajectory and the kidney-lung-heart trajectory are similar in nature to the lung-spleen-kidney axis, and problems respond well to a balance of rest and activity along with healthy dietary habits. If the patient presents with general signs of fatigue and sleep issues, it is necessary to nourish these three organs.

The Two Triads

The third set of groups is what I call triads. The triads are two groups comprising three zang organs that regulate relative excess and deficiency through the san jiao. They function to diagnose excess above with one located in the upper and middle jiao, and deficiency below with the other located in the middle and lower jiao. It is common to have to sedate the above and nourish the below when treating hot flashes. The liver plays a central role.

THE LIVER-SPLEEN-HEART TRIAD

The liver-spleen-heart triad is the three primary organs that manage the heart yang (fire) and maintain the spirit or shen. Located in the upper yang areas of the body, they are prone to excess, stagnation, and fire.

Heart fire is at the center of the hot-flash environment. The liver is yang in nature with the propensity to fire. If the stomach becomes stagnant and develops heat repletion, or if the spleen and stomach become yin deficient, they too will have the tendency of fire. Conversely, if the spleen is deficient, it cannot provide the necessary qi and blood to nourish the heart and spirit. To keep the heart fire from blazing upwards and harassing the spirit, the liver, spleen, stomach, and heart need continuous regulation. It is vital to maintain control of the fire propensity of this triad to keep the spirit calm and to quell hot flashes.

If the patient has general signs of agitation, stagnation, or fire, it is necessary to sedate these three organs. Other common menopausal-transition symptoms include insomnia, chest tightness, palpitations, and irritability or anger issues. One could say this triad is the one of fire and yang. Proper stress management and dietary habits are essential for recovery.

THE KIDNEY-LIVER-SPLEEN TRIAD

The kidney-liver-spleen triad is the three primary organs focused on generating, maintaining, and storing the essential qi (jing qi) of the body, primarily essence, blood, and yin. All of these share the same source. These organs serve as the primary source of yin and blood and have a close connection to the menstrual cycle. It is this triad that is susceptible to yin, blood, and qi deficiency from our lifestyle habits.

Yin, blood, and essence become increasingly deficient as women age. Over time, the body can begin to dry out and warm up. Therefore, it is necessary to routinely support the kidney, liver, and spleen to maintain healthy supplies. Patients with these deficiencies will tend toward nervousness, anxiety, and sleep issues. Mindfulness and proper rest are effective interventions.

Frequency, Severity, and Duration

Hot-flash symptoms can last from six months to ten years or more. The frequency, severity, and duration of all hot flashes follow a general tendency over the course of menopausal transition. From the first hot flash to the very last, they follow a curve from the initial onset to their total cessation. They start out mild early on and gradually increase, peaking in intensity at the height of menopausal transition, and then decline and eventually stop in post-menopause.

Frequency, severity, and duration ebb and flow together in unison. An increase or decrease in one is commonly seen in the others. Rating patient hot-flash frequency, severity, and duration on a mild-moderate-severe scale helps in Chinese-medicine diagnosis and tracking the clinical efficacy of acupuncture and herbal medicine treatments.

Frequency

Frequency measures how often the patient experiences hot flashes during a 24-hour period. A question about this will be easy for some to answer, while others may find it difficult.

Some women only experience hot flashes around a specific part of the day, such as during the evening or during sleep. They may even be able to say that two or three hot flashes awaken them per night. Others who have been experiencing hot flashes for a long time may experience many throughout the daytime and evening. It may be difficult for them to answer because there are too many to count.

The practitioner needs to know the overall hot-flash consistency throughout the 24-hour period. Is the patient only experiencing them during a certain time period such as morning or evening, or are they consistent throughout the day? How often is the patient experiencing hot flashes? Are they consistent and rhythmic or are they more erratic and infrequent? This information will give the clinician a better understanding of the underlying Chinese-medicine pattern.

The specific number is not clinically relevant. What is important is to see a noticeable decrease in frequency through the course of treatment.

The time of day that hot flashes occur and their overall daily rhythm are specific to each pattern type. For example, traditional yin deficiency hot flashes will present in the evening time. They will start out mild and gradually increase in frequency for a duration of time and then taper off.

Hyperactive yang qi hot flashes will be more pronounced in the morning time. They will ebb and flow throughout the rest of the day and night, spiking during times of deficiency.

Due to a myriad of reasons, qi stagnation hot flashes will present at any time or irregular times of day. Each day will be different in frequency. Clusters of hot flashes will surface and then abruptly cease.

Heat repletion hot flashes will present consistently throughout the day. They gradually increase and decrease, but never really cease.

Qi deficiency hot flashes will present at any time during the 24-hour period. They can interfere with the building of yang qi and exacerbate hot flashes in the morning hours. Much like their qi stagnation hot-flash counterpart, they too are not always consistent and will come and go unpredictably.

Blood deficiency hot flashes will present as a mild and consistent warmth throughout the day with a gradual increase during the afternoon and evening. It is common for yin deficiency and blood deficiency hot flashes to occur simultaneously.

Severity

Severity measures the strength and intensity of each individual hot flash. The severity of the hot flash can be consistent from one to the next, or may gradually increase and decrease over a period of time throughout the 24-hour period, coinciding with frequency.

Over time, severity steadily increases and then gradually declines in conjunction with the progression of menopausal transition. In some cases, severity will steadily increase over time.

In some cases, severe hot flashes will continue to be experienced well into the sixties or seventies. These exceptions are due to yang exuberance and yin burnout.

Women usually do not start out with intense hot flashes at the initial onset of menopausal transition. There are two exceptions to this rule. A total hysterectomy and bilateral salpingo-oophorectomy may generate immediate and sometimes intense hot flashes. An acute or severe disruption of qi within the body generating heat repletion can also result in intense hot flashes. This is sometimes seen in perimenopause patients and is not the result of actual menopausal transition.

Certain times of the day can present with an increase in severity. *Sunrise and morning time* are common times for women to experience a spike in hot-flash intensity. This is because the yang qi is building and increasing within the body. Along with the building of the yang qi, the blood leaves the liver and begins to circulate. Both yang qi and blood, as they become active, raise the body temperature. Together, the two create a rush to the surface of heat.

It is difficult to control this rush, especially if the yuan qi and yin essence are weak. Not only do the yuan qi and yin essence control and subdue the rushing energy of yang qi and blood, but they also cool down their fire tendencies.

Although not as common, there can be spike tendencies in hot-flash severity at *noontime*. This is the zenith of yang qi, or yang within yang. It is also the time for the heart in zangfu circadian rhythm. Excessive yang qi will exacerbate the heart fire, and some women experience particularly intense hot flashes at this time. This is an imbalance of a fire and water situation where the yang qi is excessive or the yin essence is weak.

Late afternoon and *early evening* are other times when hot flashes may increase in severity. Two patterns can create this condition. The first is a heat repletion pattern. This is a traditional "chao re" pattern, described in the *Shang Han Lun*. Based on the heavenly stems and earthly branches, it is the time (3–5pm) when the rich qi and blood of the yangming becomes effulgent and heat rushes forth. Though not as common, women with chronic digestive issues, constipation, or a history of consistent stress or unresolved emotional issues may experience a particularly intense surge of hot flashes during this time.

The second late afternoon and early evening pattern is due to blood deficiency. Blood is yin in nature and cooling for the body. As previously discussed, by the time women reach menopausal transition there is a natural tendency for the yin and blood to be deficient. Throughout the day, yin and blood resources are slowly consumed and the body will run hot. Although not as intense as a yang excess or heat repletion pattern, blood deficiency hot flashes will increase in intensity at this time.

Nighttime is by far the most common time for women to experience hot flashes. Starting around bedtime and lasting throughout the night until sunrise, hot-flash severity steadily increases to reach a pinnacle of intensity just after midnight and then gradually decreases. This is the traditional yin deficiency menopausal-transition pattern.

Midnight is the time when yin reaches its peak. Nighttime is the time for the regeneration of yin. Long uninterrupted sleep is crucial for the generation of a new healthy supply of yin. There are two factors during this time, pertaining to the balance of yin and yang that generate hot flashes.

The first factor is one of deficient yin. When the yin is weak, it loses its anchoring ability to contain the yang qi at night. As a result, the ascending and wandering nature of yang qi floats to the surface, creating hot flashes. These hot flashes usually start out mild but can become severe as menopausal transition progresses and the overall yin supply is depleted.

The second factor takes place within the regeneration of yin. The body needs yang (fire) to generate new yin (water). When this takes place during the night, the yang fire can burn excessively, generating bursts of heat that rise to the surface.

The most common time for women to experience the most problematic and severe hot flashes is 1–3am. This is the time of the liver in zangfu circadian rhythm. The liver governs the balance of yin and yang. During this time of yin regeneration, the yang qi of the liver will robustly ascend if the yin is not sufficient, thus generating severe hot flashes. Concurrent qi stagnation and heat repletion patterns will amplify this situation.

Duration

The duration measures how long each hot flash lasts and the time between hot flashes. The common duration for a hot flash is one to three minutes, followed by the cool-down and sweating period. The duration of some hot flashes may only be 30 seconds, while at the other extreme, some can last for five minutes or longer. Hot-flash duration follows the cues of frequency and severity. The increase in either or both will increase the duration of the hot flashes.

The primary concerns for many women are how severe the hot flashes and accompanying menopausal-transition symptoms will be and how long they will last. The frequency, severity, and duration are largely determined by constitution and lifestyle habits. Routine daily activity, rest, healthy dietary choices, stress management and emotional stability, and overall happiness equate to a healthier internal environment that is more resistant to problematic hot flashes.

A woman who works long hours, gets little rest, has a poor diet, exercises infrequently, and suffers from stress and emotional instability will experience more severe symptoms over a longer period of time due to the damaging nature of her lifestyle choices on her body. Conversely, a woman who lives a more balanced lifestyle of work and rest, follows a good diet and exercise plan, employs stress reduction, and whose emotions are stable will experience milder symptoms and a shorter menopausal-transition duration.

Hot Flashes and the Time of Day

Diagnosing the underlying hot-flash pattern based on the time of day in which they present is a precarious undertaking that requires several pieces of information. Simply diagnosing the hot flash based on the time of day is not completely reliable.

Chapter 18, Camp [Qi] and Guard [Qi]—Generation and Meeting, of the *Neijing Lingshu* states:

> The major yin [qi] control the interior. The major yang [qi] control the exterior. They pass through 25 units each, divided by day and night. Midnight is the yin apex. After midnight the yin weakens. At dawn the yin [qi] are exhausted and the yang [conduits] receive the qi. At noon the yang has reached its apex. When the sun is in the West, the yang [qi] weaken. When the sun goes down, the yang [qi] are exhausted and the yin [conduits] receive the qi. At midnight there is a grand meeting. All the people are asleep. That is called "link up of the yin [qi]". At dawn the yin [qi] are exhausted and the yang [conduits] receive the qi. This continues without end. It is the same set-up as that of heaven and earth. (Unschuld 2016a, p.261)

Hot flashes come and go at regular or irregular intervals and change in severity, frequency, and duration throughout the 24-hour period. Deficiency, excess, and stagnations cause hot flashes to manifest or subside at different times of the day. Clinically, I find hot flashes can flare to a four-hour cycle of qi at: 3am, 7am, 11am, 3pm, 7pm, 11pm.

Understanding the flow of the wei qi through the 24-hour cycle and the balance of yin and yang plays a major role. The relative strength and circulation of qi and blood, as well as the channel system presentation throughout the circadian clock, also play a role.

A practical understanding of these aspects of qi throughout the 24-hour cycle will help explain the pathogenesis and provide better diagnosis of the hot-flash environment.

Yin and Yang

The same chapter of the *Neijing Lingshu* states: "They circulate without stop. After 50 [circulations] a grand meeting happens. Yin and yang

[qi] penetrate each other's realm. This is like a ring without end" (Unschuld 2016a, p.260).

There is a fine and delicate balance between the yin and yang during menopausal transition. Yin and yang, along with our essence, slowly decline over time as we age. The disruption and ceasing of the menstrual cycle comes with the decline of essence. The yin and yang have to work harder to maintain balance in women during this time of life. In the clinical setting, typical menopausal-transition symptoms, including hot flashes, are commonly seen as a result of this imbalance.

Hot flashes can occur at any time of day. Some women experience more hot flashes during the nighttime, some experience the worst hot flashes in the morning, while others will experience consistent hot flashes throughout the day. With an understanding of the yin and yang cycle and time of day within the body, the practitioner can utilize this information to help diagnose why hot flashes are most prevalent at a specific time of day.

Yin and Yang Pathogenesis

The yin and yang balance is the main pathogenesis behind hot flashes. Their imbalance is reflected in the magnitude and frequency of the hot flash and is marked by the times of day at which they are at their worst and best.

Traditionally, hot flashes are noted as a yin deficiency with heat implications. This heat coming through as a hot flash is more notable during times when the relative yin is depleted. Relative, or daily, yin depletion happens steadily over time throughout the day.

Much like a car radiator running low on water after long travel on a hot day, the body runs low on yin throughout the course of the day. The body, just like a radiator, "heats up" when the coolant is low. This typically happens during the evening and nighttime when hot flashes are more prevalent.

Over time, a true yin deficiency constitution is created. It becomes increasingly difficult for the body to replenish yin during nighttime sleep. This leads to starting the new day with lower yin supplies than normal and the creation of a vicious cycle of yin depletion.

As yin depletion develops, yang qi slowly becomes unabated and has the natural ability to rouse and heat up the body. When this stage is reached, hot flashes begin to appear more frequently throughout the daytime as well.

As this imbalance further progresses and the yang becomes clearly more abundant and unabated, the yang excess will create more intense hot flashes throughout the day.

For instance, yang energy builds and rises from midnight until noon. Women with yang excess tend to have more intense hot flashes at night with increased sleep difficulty and pronounced morning and daytime hot flashes.

Wei Qi

The wei qi (guard qi or defensive qi) follows a natural-flow 24-hour cycle where it rises to the surface to warm and protect the body during the daytime and returns to the deeper regions of the zangfu organs for rejuvenation during the nighttime. The wei qi rises and falls along with our sleep cycle. The wei qi is a clock.

Chapter 76, The Movements of the Guard Qi, of the *Neijing Lingshu* states:

> The movement of the guard qi completes fifty circulations during one day and one night. During day time they move through the yang realm and complete 25 circulations. During the night they move through the yin realm and complete 25 circulations. The circulation includes the five long-term depots. (Unschuld 2016a, p.701)

Further, Chapter 18 states:

> The guard qi pass through the yin [conduits] covering 25 units. They pass through the yang [conduits] covering another 25 units, divided by day and night. (Unschuld 2016a, p.260)

Wei qi is yang, and ying qi (nutritive qi) is its yin counterpart. They balance one another and together they are the yin and yang aspects of the zhen qi. The strength of the wei qi is controlled by the overall strength of the zhen qi.

It is the overall strength of the zhen qi and the balance of the yin and yang qi that keep the wei qi coursing throughout the day. Imbalance will affect the wei qi.

At daybreak, the wei qi flows upwards and outwards to the yang realm where it provides warmth and protection for the body. It is said that once the wei qi leaves the yin realm, the eyes will open. Hot flashes can be more pronounced in the morning time when the wei qi makes its initial ascent.

At sunset, the wei qi returns back to the yin realm where it is rejuvenated within the zangfu organs. It is said that once the wei qi returns to the yin realm, the eyes will close. However, if the ying qi is not strong enough, it will be unable to harness the wei qi. The wei qi will remain in the exterior during the course of the night, where its gentle warming yang nature will generate hot flashes.

This further explains traditional nighttime hot flashes. Proper treatment is to nourish the yin aspect of the zhen qi, which is achieved by nourishing the zangfu organs in charge of the generation of the zhen qi—mainly the lung-spleen-kidney axis.

Women with general ying qi deficiency issues, including blood, will likely experience hot flashes in the evening. Conversely, women with general yang excess will also feel hot flashes in the morning and throughout the day.

The Times of Day

The yin and yang ebb and flow, rise and fall daily within the body. One turns into the other, balancing the other's increase and decline in strength. The 24-hour cycle can be broken into four main yin and yang sections as described in this passage from the *Neijing*:

> Hence it is said: In yin is yin; in yang is yang. From dawn to noon, this is the yang of heaven; it is the yang in the yang. From noon to dusk, this is the yang of heaven; it is the yin in the yang. From early evening to the crowing of the cocks, this is the yin of heaven; it is the yin in the yin. From the crowing of the cocks to dawn, this is the yin of heaven; it is the yang in the yin. (Unschuld and Tessenow 2011, pp.36–39)

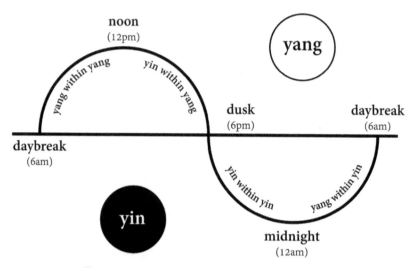

FIGURE 5.2: 24-HOUR FLOW OF YIN AND YANG

6am–12pm (yang within yang)
12pm–6pm (yin within yang)
6pm–12am (yin within yin)
12am–6am (yang within yin)

Midnight is ultimate yin. It is the time when the yang qi begins to build—the time of yang within yin. Blood has not yet left the liver to flow back into the channels. Yang qi will become strong and rise too early if yin is weak or deficient. Wei qi will float if the blood is weak and cannot harness it. If this happens, there will be pulses of heat soon after midnight and women will experience hot flashes in the early morning hours.

At *daybreak*, the yang builds and grows ever stronger. Our eyes open from sleep as we enter the yang within yang stage. This is when the overall dominance of yin qi transitions to the yang qi. Yang qi will gain too much momentum as it builds if yin is deficient or yang is excessive. It is also the time when blood is released from the liver and surges through the channels, and an abundance of wei qi is released. This causes strong bursts of heat and is why some women experience intense hot flashes at this time.

At the peak of *midday*, the sun is at its hottest and yang has reached its zenith. Yang begins to wane and yin begins to grow. It is the time of yin within yang. If the yang qi is extreme, women will have consistent hot flashes throughout the daytime. Yin and blood show signs of weakness over the course of the day. If this happens, there is an overall rise in heat.

Sunset is the time of yin within yin. There is less yang and wei qi activity as they wane and begin their descent into yin and blood. It is now the time for yin to build and grow in strength. It is when the overall dominance of yang qi transitions to the yin qi. If yin is weak and unable to lead fire downwards, or if the yang is effulgent, there will be mild bursts of heat and women tend to have evening hot flashes.

Blood deficiency tidal fever case study: A 38-year-old female patient presented with mild to moderate afternoon hot flashes that began after the delivery of her second child two months previous. The hot flashes started in the afternoon and abated in the evening. The patient had a history of celiac disease and presented with low appetite, gas, bloating, loose stools, and mild nausea. She had recently lost her father and had grief and stress, low lactation, and mild chest tightness. The patient had a history of nightly nightmares and night sweats since childhood. Her pulse was deep, thin, and slightly rapid. Her tongue was slightly pale, with no coating, and with a slight tremor.

I originally diagnosed this patient with spleen and kidney deficiency, qi stagnation, and deficiency fire. I used a general hot-flash deficiency acupuncture prescription and added KI2 and PC6. After the first acupuncture treatment, her hot flashes and nausea increased for one day and then decreased for two days. The patient described her hot flashes as having a "moving feeling" within that I describe as the ebb and flow of tidal fever. Her lactation worsened, with less milk production, yet she experienced no nightmares for two days. I observed that the patient was slightly pale.

Afternoon tidal fever is commonly the result of yangming excess or blood deficiency. The symptoms obviously pointed to blood deficiency. I changed my strategy for the second acupuncture treatment and switched my focus to the chong mai and nourishing the sea of blood. I added ST37 and ST39, subtracted SP6 and added SP4, and added LU9 and SI1. After the second treatment, the patient's hot flashes and nausea were exacerbated for one day and then completely disappeared. The patient's lactation improved, her digestion and energy improved with less loose stools, and she was experiencing less nightmares. The patient completed a final third acupuncture treatment and reported feeling much better.

Circadian Clock

The Chinese-medicine twelve-channel circadian clock is a conglomeration of classical theory and highlights the flow of the ying qi through the channel system. There are many hot-flash connections to be made that can help strengthen hot-flash diagnosis based on time of day, yin and yang, ying and wei qi, and zangfu organs.

3–5am: The Lung Channel of Hand Taiyin
5–7am: The Large Intestine Channel of Hand Yangming
7–9am: The Stomach Channel of Foot Yangming
9–11am: The Spleen Channel of Foot Taiyin

The first circuit of qi flows through the taiyin and yangming channels. The taiyin (greater yin) channels belong to the lung and spleen. The lung and spleen are the two chief zangfu organs in charge of generating qi. They are the two zang organs most susceptible to deficiency. The yangming (yang brightness) channels belong to the large intestine and stomach. They are the two channels and fu organs rich in qi and blood and susceptible to "brightness" or exuberance.

Ying qi (yin) and wei qi (yang) are components of the true (zhen) qi. When there is an overall qi deficiency within the body, there will be a yin and yang disruption in the balance between the ying and wei qi. An overall qi deficiency can weaken the ying qi and allow the wei qi to be unopposed. Unopposed wei qi during the morning has the tendency to flow excessively outwards to the surface, creating hot flashes.

Conversely, when qi (yang) becomes overabundant, whether due to stagnation or heat repletion, the yangming channels will become excessive. The large intestine and stomach fu organs are susceptible to repletion patterns. Yangming repletion, as previously discussed, will generate tidal heat effusion. Yangming repletion can cause hot flashes, with possible intensity during these times.

11am–1pm: The Heart Channel of Hand Shaoyin
1–3pm: The Small Intestine Channel of Hand Taiyang
3–5pm: The Urinary Bladder Channel of Foot Taiyang
5–7pm: The Kidney Channel of Foot Shaoyin

The second circuit of qi flows through the shaoyin and taiyang channels. The shaoyin (lesser yin) channels belong to the heart and kidney. The heart and kidney are the two chief organs in charge of the fire and water balance within the body. They are the two organs mainly in charge of the hot-flash environment. The taiyang (greater yang) channels belong to the small intestine and urinary bladder. They are the two main channels in charge of bringing yang qi to the surface. As in the name, the taiyang channels have great ability to control yang qi and the yang areas of the body.

The hot-flash environment depends on the balance of the heart and kidney. The potential for hot flashes increases when the fire becomes excessive or the water becomes deficient. The heart sits at high noon. There is a greater potential for hot flashes at this time if the heart fire becomes excessive.

As stated, the taiyang channels, are in charge of bringing yang qi to the surface to warm and protect the body. Taiyang will become "greater" than normal if yin becomes exhausted and yang cannot descend, or if the yang is excessive. The abundant yang qi will continue to stay at the surface. Even though this illustrates a common yin and yang imbalance, its influence on the taiyang channels can cause hot flashes during this time.

On the other side of the water-fire equilibrium, the kidney holds its position at dusk, and this is the time when yang is transitioning over to yin. If the yin water is weak and unable to descend, the yang fire stays at the surface and in the upper regions of the body. This unopposed fire during the evening is the classic clinical hot-flash scenario.

7–9pm: The Pericardium Channel of Hand Jueyin
9–11pm: The San Jiao Channel of Hand Shaoyang
11pm–1am: The Gallbladder of Foot Shaoyang
1–3am: The Liver Channel of Foot Jueyin

The third circuit of qi flows through the jueyin and shaoyang channels. The jueyin (pivoting yin) channels belong to the pericardium and liver. These two channels serve as the "pivot" between yin and yang, hence the time of day. The shaoyang (lesser yang) channels belong to the san jiao and gallbladder. They are the two channels associated with and that regulate the exterior (yang) and interior (yin) areas of the body. As with other yang channels, they are susceptible to excess.

The jueyin channels and zang organs are the yang within yin, or the fire within the water. They have an active role at controlling and regulating the yin and yang within the body. They are susceptible to yang excess due to stagnation, repletion patterns, and yin and blood deficiency.

Along with their jueyin counterparts, the shaoyang channels play an active role in controlling and regulating qi flow and yin and yang within the body. This is particularly noticeable during the times of day when one turns over to the other, especially at midnight, daybreak, noon, and dusk.

When the jueyin and shaoyang are affected, they lose their regulatory abilities over yin and yang. Once both sets of channels are disrupted, hot flashes will be pronounced during this time and more erratic, frequent, or intense throughout the 24-hour period.

Respiration—Balance of the Lung and Kidney

Balanced breath work is the cornerstone of meditation, longevity, and overall health. Respiration is able to reestablish nervous and endocrine system coherence, and these are the two primary systems involved in the hot-flash environment.

The lung and kidney relationship is in itself the great qi regulator of the body. Balanced and uninterrupted, effortlessly coming and going, rising and falling; together, the lung and kidney push and pull the tides within the body, the tides of yin and yang, blood, essence, and qi.

As stated in Chapter 1, inhalation is yin and exhalation is yang. Our breath works like a great bellows, continually generating and moving qi and blood throughout the body. Upon inhalation, the lung (taiyin) gathers the air (da qi) within it and in turn the kidney (shaoyin) grasps hold of it and leads the qi downwards to receive it. Within the kidney, the air qi combines with the essential (jing) qi. Upon exhalation, the movement is reversed. The kidney releases the newly engendered qi upwards to combine with the food and drink (gu qi) within the spleen (taiyin) to create the source (yuan) qi, which arrives back in the chest where it becomes the true (zhen) qi. This principle is what I call the "axis of life" or the lung-spleen-kidney axis. This axis is of utmost importance, for the inhalation and exhalation of the breath generates and circulates qi and blood.

Balancing Water and Fire

The lung and kidney mechanics work alongside the water and fire (yin and yang) exchange between the heart and kidney. This dual system controls excitation and calmness in the following ways.

Traditionally, inhaling qi descends to the kidney and exhaling qi ascends to the lung, benefiting the parasympathetic nervous system, which is considered yin in nature. This normal abdominal breath descends the fire (yang) from the heart to the kidney and ascends the water (yin) from the kidney back up to the heart.

When the traditional breath is reversed with the inhalation intention into the lung and exhalation intention into the kidney, it benefits the sympathetic nervous system, which is considered yang in nature. This alteration of breath ascends the fire (yang) from the kidney to the heart and descends water (yin) from the heart to the kidney.

These breathing techniques can be used for the stimulation of yin and yang. It depends on the particular person and situation whether one or the other is required.

The Diaphragm and Qi Stagnation

General qi stagnation cuts off the inhalation to the kidney and exhalation to the lung. Qi stagnation particularly affects the shaoyang (san jiao and gallbladder) and jueyin (pericardium and liver) channels that traverse the chest, ribs, diaphragm, and abdomen.

When these channels are affected by the flow of qi, they have the tendency to create muscle tightness in these areas. Qi stagnation and muscle tightness will cause shallow, short, difficult, or hasty breathing.

Over time, the lung loses its ability to govern qi, disrupting the heart's ability to govern blood. The result is the decline of qi and blood circulation throughout the zangfu organs and the entire body.

At the same time, the descending qi will stop at the level of the liver and will not reach the kidney. The kidney becomes cut off from receiving vital qi and will go into premature decline. While over-compensating, the liver will gradually become excessive in yang and deficient of yin and blood, and lose its ability to balance yin and yang qi throughout the body. This mirrors dysregulation within the HPO axis.

The normal aging process is accelerated if the inadequate govern-ance of qi and blood is not remedied and if the vital qi is not able to descend to the kidney. An early menopausal transition and a myriad of systemic issues will eventually arise, leading to chronic disease.

Resolving qi stagnation leads to regaining proper breath, which in turn reestablishes qi and blood circulation, yin and yang balance, heat dissipation, and the lung and kidney reestablishment.

The Creation of Stagnation

Stagnation is largely the result of a sedentary lifestyle, dietary irregular-ities, or emotional discord stemming from the seven affects (joy, anger, anxiety, thought, sorrow, fear, and fright). As qi stagnation develops over time, the body begins to modify its physiological mechanisms around it. Chest and diaphragm muscles lose their ability to flex and contract because qi and blood can no longer nourish and freely cir-culate. Normal respiration is disrupted, causing irregular breathing habits. The results are shortness of breath and shallow, labored, or staggered breathing, along with frequent yawning, sighing, and the need for gulps and deep breaths.

This explains why exercise helps some people who are experiencing qi stagnation. Exercise helps return the breathing to a normal state. It is interesting to note, however, that if activity and emotional patterns are not changed, when exercise ceases, the breathing issues return. Once the breath is disrupted and the muscles are not freely functioning, the situation progresses, affecting the heart rate and heartbeat. This in turn will lead to qi and blood circulation issues and further spirit issues involving the heart, including sleep disorders and anxiety.

Diagnosing the Breath

Inspecting the patient's breath provides valuable insight into the patient's overall state of health. One key concept for diagnosing the breath is to see if the patient has any labored, short, or shallow breathing. This can easily be seen when the patient walks through the clinic door, is sitting across from you, or is on the treatment table.

Notice if the patient has trouble speaking and breathing at the same time. Do they struggle to catch their breath? When they are breathing, do they only breathe into their chest and take small short breaths?

If this is so, the first and most basic treatment a practitioner can initiate is to start opening up their kidney and lung qi. Opening up this gateway releases pent-up stagnation and allows the qi to flow to the zangfu organs. Qi, blood, and body fluids will all regain their natural flow and the patient will be able to regain health.

If the lung and kidney qi flow is not addressed, it will be difficult to gain any sustaining and lasting benefit from treatment. It is best to teach the patient how to breathe into their abdomen and how to control movement of their diaphragm while on the treatment table. Rest the palm of your hand on their upper abdomen as they breathe. Show them how to breathe deeply into the abdomen where your hand is by, taking long and even inhalations and exhalations.

Conclusion

In Chinese medicine, proper breath balances the lung and kidney and in turn balances the lung and heart ability to govern qi and blood throughout the body, thus reestablishing the water and fire balance between the heart and kidney. This is how proper respiration can treat hot flashes.

Some hot-flash patients experience good results with minimal help from a practitioner by applying these basic principles. By changing lifestyle habits, including meditation and yoga to help bond breath and body, they experience significant relief from problematic hot flashes. A patient's breath is their life source and one of the most basic ways to generate and maintain qi throughout the body.

Temperature and Tolerance

Hot-flash patients experience rushes of heat. As already discussed, they have many causes. As acupuncturists and Chinese-medicine practitioners, it is necessary that we know the source in order to treat the hot flash effectively.

Diagnosing a patient's aversion to, acceptance of, and tolerance for temperature is very useful in the clinic. It assists in understanding if the patient has a general excess or deficient hot-flash environment. It is true that the hot-flash environment is regularly an excess/deficiency state.

Simple diagnostic questions about temperature are helpful in looking beyond the surface symptoms and into the root of the patient's true foundation.

Deficiency Patterns

It is common for hot-flash patients to have yin and blood deficiency, or perhaps even qi and yang deficiency, with concurrent deficiency heat or stagnation and heat repletion.

The root pattern is deficiency. Even though these patients are experiencing hot flashes and waves of uncomfortable heat, which seem excess in nature, beneath the surface is weakness and vacuity. These patients will love warm and dislike cold weather. This is because the deficiency needs warmth. They may even say that they are always cold. Simply asking if the patient enjoys summer, enjoys the sun and outdoors, and enjoys the warm weather will give the practitioner a lot of diagnostic information.

Excess Patterns

In contrast, there are patients with excess fire, yin fire, stagnated heat, or phlegm-fire. These derive from excess. It is common for these patients to present with deficiency symptoms as well. It can be difficult to be certain which came first—the deficiency generating the excess state, or the excess state consuming vital qi and presenting with deficiency symptoms. Again, asking questions about temperature preference and tolerance will lead the practitioner to the root of how to address treatment. Excess patients will generally prefer cooler weather and air conditioning, and may even sleep with a fan or with the window open.

Excess patients may also present with generalized irritability and intolerances. They may seem both physically and mentally uncomfortable. Clearing the excess will relieve some of the symptoms. If these symptoms are intractable and do not respond to treatment, this points to a deeper shen disturbance.

Some patients will mention a dislike for hot and humid weather. This is not typically a useful indication of deficiencies or excess. Most people simply find hot and humid weather uncomfortable.

Cold Extremities

Hot-flash patients, whether excess or deficient, may present with cold fingers and toes. This symptom does not give the practitioner much added information to assist in the overall diagnosis, for several reasons.

First, with age comes deficiency of the vital qi. Vital qi, over time, slowly loses its ability to flow to the ends of the extremities to provide warmth. Second, generalized stress and anxiety are common in modern life. This can generate stagnation and impair the flow of qi and blood in reaching the extremities to provide warmth. Third, excess can gather within the interior and generate stagnation and heat repletion patterns. These excess yang patterns prevent the yang qi from making its ways to the ends of the extremities to provide warmth. This is called a true heat false cold pattern in Chinese medicine. Finally, women during menopausal transition can have a decline of kidney yin and yang. Here, the chong mai is deficient and susceptible to yang qi and stagnation influences. This can generate ascending yin deficiency heat with descending yang deficiency cold. This is why menopausal-transition patients experience hot flashes yet have cold extremities.

Cold fingers and toes are often due to a combination of age, stress, stagnation, deficiency, or excess. This leads us back to the original question: does the patient enjoy the warm weather? Those with true deficiency will respond with "Yes." These patients will especially enjoy acupuncture treatments with heat lamps, while the excess patient will have an aversion to the use of direct heat lamps or a warmer treatment room.

Conclusion

The tolerance of heat and cold is a very useful tool in diagnosing the hot-flash environment. It also presents a useful opportunity to talk to and explain our understanding of the hot-flash environment to the patient.

Treatment may or may not affect a patient's preference for heat or cold. Most often, excess patients will always have a heat intolerance. Likewise, deficient patients may always have an aversion to cooler temperatures. These preferences may be partly due to genetics and partly due to lifestyle habits.

Patient Initial Health Intake

The patient initial health intake gathers abundant necessary information about the patient's past and current health situation. The information gathered in this intake gives the practitioner insight into the internal medical realm of the patient.

The intake protocol supports the practitioner in two ways: it organizes all the necessary questions to prevent inadvertent omissions, and provides a record to refer back to during the treatment process. Without a protocol, intakes can be too long and unfocused.

Most importantly, the initial health intake is a patient map. Experienced clinicians see connections among the patient answers that support a Chinese-medicine pattern and clinical diagnosis.

In many cases, the information gathered in the intake will suffice in making an initial diagnosis. Questioning the patient, taking the pulse, and observing the tongue should serve to verify and clarify the clinician's diagnosis.

Clinically diagnosing hot flashes seems easy at first. However, the true hot-flash environment pattern may not be revealed until after several acupuncture treatments, giving way to a treatment-confirmed diagnosis. The practitioner must have patience.

Patient Health History

The patient health history consists of mandatory questions to help protect both the patient and the healthcare provider. Written and verbal answers to certain questions are medical red flags; it is up to the practitioner to be familiar with them. Patients may need to seek immediate medical care or be referred to their primary care physician.

The responses in this section are routinely helpful in understanding the patient's past and current conditions and provide evidence that may have influence on the hot-flash environment.

CURRENT TREATMENTS, THERAPIES, MEDICATIONS, SUPPLEMENTS, AND HERBAL FORMULAS

Patients partaking in preventative healthcare measures is generally a positive sign. This can include both physical and internal therapies. Preventative care does have its limitations. There can be too much of a good thing. Pay special attention to making sure that the patient is not overdoing any one particular or multiple treatments, especially herbs and supplements. Overdoing equals overdose and may in fact be detrimental to the patient's overall health.

Patient answers may also reveal potential problems and health concerns, especially if they are taking prescription medications. Ask questions about the reasons and need for taking them. Are they necessary to treat an underlying condition, or are they treating a symptom?

The difficulty in treating patients increases if they are taking multiple prescriptions. The more medications they are taking, the more possible drug interactions and potential side effects must be considered as potential causes for symptoms. Patients in this category have the tendency to respond slowly to acupuncture treatments. It may also be necessary to forego herbal medicine due to adverse drug-herb interactions.

ALLERGIES

Allergies in patients are most often a pre-heaven (kidney) qi or post-heaven (lung and spleen) qi deficiency issue. While some people are born with food or environmental allergies, others have a tendency to develop them over time, including adult onset and age-related allergies.

In many cases, allergies are the result of a constitutional weakness. A change in climate, activity, and dietary habits can improve the patient's overall health and be the deciding factor in whether or not the patient continues to experience allergies.

Practitioners must look closely at the patient's diet and the strength of their digestion. Many people in today's society develop allergies because of qi deficient digestion, lack of activity, stress, and dietary choices. This includes allergic skin disorders.

INFECTIOUS AND CHRONIC DISEASES

It is important to gather patient information on past and present disease and other severe health-related issues. It is essential to know of any current potential health risks for the patient and how they are involved in the underlying hot-flash environment.

Acupuncture and Chinese medicine are very helpful in supporting chronically ill patients and in the rehabilitation process following a severe illness. It is ethically necessary to know the possible risks for severe and chronic disease. Some patients may require medical care above and beyond what a Chinese-medicine practitioner can provide.

These illnesses include cancer, diabetes, hepatitis, infectious disease, high blood pressure, seizures, stroke, HIV/AIDS, respiratory infections, chronic obstructive pulmonary disorder (COPD), pneumonia, hemophilia, blood-clotting issues, sexually transmitted diseases (STDs), tuberculosis, multiple sclerosis, dementia, and cirrhosis.

Acute, chronic, or severe disease will have an impact on the body's vital qi, blood, essence, and yin and yang. Whether it's severe depletion, repletion, or stagnation, any imbalances of this nature can directly or indirectly cause or amplify the hot-flash environment. The practitioner must consider these factors when treating these patients.

Patient Lifestyle History

Patient lifestyle-history questions focus primarily on the patient's exercise activity and dietary habits. These have a direct influence on the lung-spleen-kidney axis and the patient's constitution.

It is vital to know if the patient's current constitution has the ability to generate and provide essential qi and blood for their overall health and recovery. If it does not, it is necessary to start by improving the constitution. If a weakened constitution is not addressed, symptoms will return following treatments, even when the patient initially shows improvement.

The simple process of answering the questions on paper can have a positive effect on a patient. It may help them make the connection between their lifestyle choices and their overall health constitution. When a patient cognitively makes this link, they will begin to understand their role in the healing process.

WEIGHT

It may be obvious if the patient is overweight or underweight when they enter the clinic. It is short-sighted to diagnosis thin patients with a yin or blood deficient pattern and heavyset patients with a yin excess and deficient pattern. Weight doesn't necessarily dictate the hot-flash pattern. Even if a patient is underweight or overweight, they may have a healthy or unhealthy constitution. It is useful to know how the patient sees themselves, and this may reveal useful clinical information about their overall spirit.

EXERCISE HABITS

Daily physical activity is critical to good health. Too much or a lack of activity and exercise will have a detrimental effect on the constitution. Over time, excessive amounts of activity will consume the vital qi, whereas a sedentary lifestyle cannot produce enough vital qi. Activity and exercise habits develop over a lifetime and are difficult to change.

It is valuable for the practitioner to ask about the frequency and intensity of a patient's activities and what they enjoy doing.

Overactivity case study: A 55-year-old female patient presented with extreme hot flashes and night sweating for two to three years. The hot-flash frequency was every 40 minutes. Accompanying symptoms included insomnia with frequent waking due to hot flashes and severe physical and mental fatigue. Her pulse was moderate and her tongue was puffy and pale, and had a white coating.

The original diagnosis was kidney and liver yin deficiency with deficiency heat. I used a general hot-flash deficiency acupuncture prescription. The patient underwent three weeks of acupuncture treatments that improved her symptoms by 60%. The relief plateaued from there and after ten treatments in total her hot flashes began fluctuating from mild to severe without control.

Upon reevaluation, the patient talked about how on weekends she went on long-distance bike rides. There was a pattern showing that the patient responded better to treatments when she didn't go on any long-distance bike rides at the previous weekend. I recommended the patient decreased her overall biking distances and only went for long distances once per month. The patient decreased her mileage and took more weekends off from biking. The results were remarkable. The patient's hot flashes dramatically reduced, along with her other symptoms. She was astonished to learn that she was able to control her hot flashes this way. The conclusion is that exercise is positive and an important health habit, but excessive exercise depletes the vital qi, which allows qi and yang to ascend and harass the heart fire.

DIET AND DIETARY HABITS

This area arguably has a substantial impact on our overall health. It is the area where the patient has the greatest control. It is also the area that has the greatest potential for problems.

There are many types of diets including carnivore, vegetarian, vegan, paleo, low-carbohydrate, gluten-free, low-fat, crash, detox, belief-based, and medically necessary diets. There is not one special diet that is perfect for everyone. What is healthy for some may not be healthy for others. It is important for each individual to find a healthy and well-balanced diet that works for them. This is achieved when the patient has energy throughout the day and feels good, has a clear mind, and is free of any digestive issues.

Cleaning up a poor diet is a good first step for any patient. Some useful ways to do this include: eating more fruits and vegetables, reducing meat intake, limiting the amount of simple carbohydrates and favoring complex carbohydrates and whole grains, improving hydration, and avoiding fast foods, processed foods, and sugary foods and drinks.

Consistency is another useful dietary habit change. Overeating, undereating, skipping meals, and eating too much of the same thing will have a negative impact on the spleen and stomach's ability to generate qi and blood. The digestive tract prefers stability and reliability. It is much like workers on an assembly line who enjoy steady work and dislike being bored or overworked. Too little work and the yin within the digestive tract will burn out creating deficiency heat. Too much work creates stagnation and heat repletion.

Stomach yin deficiency case study: A 51-year-old female patient presented with severe hot flashes and night sweating for ten years. Accompanying symptoms included severe insomnia with difficulty falling asleep and frequent waking at night, physical fatigue, and severe irritability. Her pulse was thin and rapid. Her tongue was red with no coating.

The original diagnosis was kidney and liver yin deficiency, with deficiency fire. I used a general hot-flash deficiency acupuncture prescription and added KI2, LR13, and ST44. The patient underwent eight acupuncture treatments with only a 40% reduction in hot flashes. Her stress and energy responded well, while her hot flashes and sleep responded only moderately.

Upon reevaluation, it was clear the patient had a stressful job, worked long hours, skipped meals, and drank coffee and very little water. My hypothesis was that the patient's hot flashes were not responding well because her stomach yin was severely damaged due to a long history of poor eating habits. My recommendation was for her to eat regular meals, have smaller portions, keep snacks on hand, and stay hydrated. After two weeks of eating yogurt for breakfast, snacking on fruit during the day, and switching from coffee during the day to water, her hot flashes, sleep, energy, and stress issues were all reduced or eliminated.

My conclusion is that the body overheats when the stomach yin burns out, much like a car overheating when the radiator runs low on water. This type of hot flash is common. I try to pay close attention to the patients who skip meals, especially breakfast. I've treated many stomach yin deficiency hot-flash cases simply with dietary recommendations. The key is to never allow the stomach to become empty where it can overheat. I like to recommend yogurt, cantaloupe, apples, berries, lean meats, cucumbers, celery, and water. I think that 48–72 ounces per day is adequate. Patients in this category will benefit from not eating fried, processed, and heat-agitating foods, which can aggravate the stomach fire.

HYDRATION

Hydration needs to be addressed separately. Water is yin and sedates yang. Water controls fire. Low water intake and dehydration allow the yin and blood to dwindle. This allows for yang hyperactivity and a rise in heat, thus creating a hot-flash environment.

Hydration also has a direct effect on the HPO axis. Water affects the overall blood volume and circulation. If the body is dehydrated, the blood volume and circulation will decrease within the brain and throughout the body. This creates difficulty for the hormones in traveling and communicating within the HPO axis. Water has a soothing effect on the nervous system. If the body becomes dehydrated, the nervous system will tend to excitation. When this happens, the hypothalamus, in particular, will lose its ability to control thermoregulation.

Proper hydration is one of the easiest methods a patient can incorporate to ease menopausal transition and improve hot flashes. In general, one liter of water per day is a good starting suggestion that can be increased to 1.5 liters or more based on stature.

Coffee, tea, soda, juice, and alcohol do not count for proper hydration. Based on Chinese medicine, they all have a specific effect on the body. Coffee and tea are generally drying in nature. They improve qi function, yet they can consume and deplete qi and yin, creating a yang active environment. Soda and juice are tonifying based on their sweetness, but only in small quantities. They tend to create stagnation and yin excess.

Alcohol is yang in nature and has the potential to generate yang and fire within the body, especially within the liver. It is a good idea for patients to drink less of the above-mentioned beverages and replace them with water. Menopausal women who drink alcohol tend to have worse sleep issues and hot flashes. Patients can even see their hot flashes worsen at times of alcohol consumption. Many patients in this category are otherwise healthy. Patients willing to consume less alcohol, cut it out completely, or abstain for a week or two can see hot flashes improve.

Women's Health History

The menstrual cycle is a useful diagnostic tool in Chinese medicine. It is a medical record that follows the female patient throughout life from menarche to the FMP. Knowing the patient's menstrual history and tendencies lays the groundwork for understanding the individual's hot-flash environment. Diagnosing the menstrual cycle is especially useful during menopausal transition and provides necessary information about changes or fluctuations in qi and blood and yin and yang.

MENSTRUAL CYCLE HISTORY

It is good to know the age of the patient when she had her first period. The age of menarche in Western countries has declined significantly in the last 200 years, from approximately 17 years to 13 years. In Chinese medicine, this points to excess and deficient issues. On the other hand, some girls' first period is at a much later age. This can point to a pre-heaven qi issue involving essence deficiency, or perhaps a post-heaven qi issue involving blood deficiency. This information is useful in the clinic because it gives the practitioner a foundational understanding of the patient's congenital and acquired qi.

The patient's normal menstrual cycle, from late teens until menopause, provides a unique and insightful understanding of the patient's individual qi and blood, and yin and yang dynamic. Tracking any monthly changes, or lack thereof, over this long period of time provides the clinician with a bird's-eye view of the patient's overall health.

This history allows the practitioner to make comparisons between the patient's normal menstrual cycle and the changes in their cycle during menopausal transition. During transition, most women begin to experience fluctuations in their cycle. It is valuable to know what used to be normal versus the current presentation.

MENSTRUAL IRREGULARITIES

Many excess and deficiency patterns disrupt the natural menstrual cycle. It is common for women to experience abnormal disruptions due to deficiencies of qi and blood, imbalances within the yin and yang dynamic, stagnations of qi, blood, or damp-phlegm, or cold and heat generated from repletion, deficiency, or stagnation issues.

These dysfunctions interfere with the qi and blood circulation to, from, and within the uterus. Familiar results include frequent periods, early periods, heavy periods, irregular periods, spotting, bleeding between periods, or continuous bleeding. It is valuable to ask the patient about any abnormal menstrual changes. Some useful questions include:

How would you describe your current periods?

☐ Heavy periods

☐ Light periods

☐ Irregular periods

☐ Shorter periods

☐ Longer periods

☐ Frequent spotting

☐ Bleed between periods

☐ Painful periods

☐ Clots with periods

How would you describe the color of your periods?

☐ Bright red

☐ Dark red

☐ Pale red

☐ Purple red

☐ Brown red

Menopausal-transition menstrual irregularities last one to three years on average. The practitioner should inform the patient that this is completely normal. Irregularities beginning sooner than menopausal transition point to pronounced deficiency, excess, or stagnation issues and are not the norm.

Heavy, prolonged spotting or constant bleeding is a normal menopausal-transition occurrence. Many cases will naturally cease or resolve with routine acupuncture treatments or herbal medicine. Abnormal bleeding is due to combined qi deficiency, stagnation, and heat patterns.

Abnormal bleeding is a medical concern if it does not stop. In this case, it is necessary to refer the patient to see a Western medical specialist. A specialist needs to screen for and rule out endometrial cancer. Abnormal bleeding is often due to polyps, cysts, fibroids, or endometriosis complications. Contraceptives and endometrial ablations are common therapies to treat these issues.

PERIOD SYMPTOMS

Symptoms experienced during the menstrual period are also diagnostically useful in clinic. They provide additional information about the overall strength of the woman's qi and blood.

Many common period symptoms involve qi deficiency. Qi and blood are redirected to the uterus as the female body prepares for the period. The rest of the body has less overall qi and blood to work with during this time. This creates an environment in which the zangfu organs have to function with less qi and there is less qi and blood circulating through the channel system. The result is weakness and stagnation.

Premenstrual Syndrome (PMS) is a group of physical and emotional symptoms that affect most women. These symptoms can happen before, during, and after their period depending on the severity of the stagnation and the overall weakness of the qi and blood. A useful question is:

Which symptoms do you have with your period?

- ☐ Breast tenderness
- ☐ Irritability
- ☐ Sadness
- ☐ Headaches
- ☐ Fatigue
- ☐ Swelling
- ☐ Loose stools or digestive issues
- ☐ Cold and flu symptoms
- ☐ Body aches
- ☐ Acne or other skin issues

If symptoms and the underlying imbalances persist, women in this category are prone to suffer enhanced menopausal-transition issues at an earlier-than-normal age.

Diagnosing the Hot Flash

The hot flash is only one symptom women experience during menopausal transition. It is the number-one symptom women seek treatment for. In the clinical setting, there are many questions to ask and ways to track the hot flash.

The following comprehensive list covers almost every aspect of the hot-flash intake. It provides useful questions and answers that help diagnose the hot flash as a symptom. Detailed descriptions and supporting information can be found throughout the book.

Some content may be too much for some practitioners and provide little clinical support, while for others it will provide necessary and vital information for research and tracking treatment efficacy.

FAMILY HISTORY

Gathering hot-flash family history supports congenital and genetic traits. It also provides a menopausal-transition outlook for both the patient and the practitioner, as family members tend to follow similar patterns. Conversely, women who have altered their lifestyle habits from the traditional family habits may fare better or worse depending on their choices.

It is enjoyable to see and treat women who've improved their life situations and then go through menopausal transition with few issues. Questions can include:

How many siblings do you have?

Where are you in the sibling order?

How old were your parents when you were born?

Were there any complications with your birth?

Have your mother, female relatives, or siblings experienced menopausal symptoms? ☐ Yes ☐ No

If so, please specify.

GENERAL HOT-FLASH SYMPTOMS

Rate the following symptoms based on the severity: hot flashes, sweating (episodes of sweating):

☐ None

☐ Mild

☐ Moderate

☐ Severe

☐ Extremely severe

Do you experience hot flashes?	☐ Yes	☐ No
Do you experience night sweating?	☐ Yes	☐ No
Do you frequently sweat?	☐ Yes	☐ No
Do you sweat easily?	☐ Yes	☐ No
Do you get hot easy?	☐ Yes	☐ No
Do you get cold easy?	☐ Yes	☐ No
Do you only get cold after a hot flash and sweating?	☐ Yes	☐ No
Do only your fingers, toes, ears, or nose get cold?	☐ Yes	☐ No
Does your entire body get cold?	☐ Yes	☐ No
Do you enjoy the warm weather?	☐ Yes	☐ No
Do you prefer cooler temperatures?	☐ Yes	☐ No

How long have you been experiencing hot flashes?

- ☐ <1 year
- ☐ 1–3 years
- ☐ 4–5 years
- ☐ 6–10 years
- ☐ 10+ years

How frequent are your hot flashes?

- ☐ Infrequent
- ☐ 1 per hour
- ☐ 2–3 per hour
- ☐ 4–9 per hour
- ☐ 10+ per hour

How many hot flashes do you experience in 24 hours?

- ☐ 1–5
- ☐ 6–10
- ☐ 11–24
- ☐ 25+
- ☐ Constant

How long does a typical hot flash last for you?

- ☐ 1–10 seconds
- ☐ 11–30 seconds
- ☐ 31–59 seconds
- ☐ 1–2 minutes

☐ 3+ minutes

☐ Constant

When do you experience hot flashes?

☐ Mornings

☐ Afternoons

☐ Evenings

☐ During sleep

☐ Constantly

When are your hot flashes the worst?

☐ Mornings

☐ Afternoons

☐ Evenings

☐ During sleep

☐ Constantly

Do your hot flashes interfere or disrupt any parts of your lifestyle?

☐ Work

☐ Leisure

☐ Exercise

☐ Sleep

Hot flashes and heat symptoms can manifest and be felt in different locations of the body. Bursts of qi can start systemically and be felt all over the body. Some will feel a rush from the abdomen upwards followed by a sense of heat in the chest, similar to qi rising via the chong mai or running piglet qi. Other patients will feel heat begin in the chest, neck, and face. Whichever the case, documenting heat in specific areas is quite fascinating and can reveal specific patterns.

When experiencing a hot flash, do you feel heat everywhere in your body or only specific areas?

- ☐ Everywhere
- ☐ Only specific areas

Please check the specific areas where you experience heat with a hot flash:

- ☐ Head
- ☐ Face and cheeks
- ☐ Ears
- ☐ Neck and throat
- ☐ Chest
- ☐ Abdomen
- ☐ Groin and genitalia
- ☐ Neck and upper back
- ☐ Along the spine
- ☐ Lower back
- ☐ Arms and forearms
- ☐ Palms and fingers
- ☐ Upper legs
- ☐ Lower legs
- ☐ Soles of feet

Do you have any triggers for your hot flashes?

☐ Alcohol

☐ Coffee or caffeine

☐ Any hot beverages

☐ Other beverages (please specify)

☐ Dehydration

☐ Specific foods (please specify)

☐ Skipping meals

☐ Not eating enough

☐ During meals

☐ After eating

☐ Exercise or activity

☐ Fatigue

☐ Working long hours

☐ Sleep

☐ Warm environment

☐ Cool environment

☐ Air conditioning

☐ Humidity

☐ Sunlight

☐ Wind

☐ Stress or irritability

☐ Worry or depression

Do you experience any peculiar or specific
sensations before the start of a hot flash? ☐ Yes ☐ No

If yes, please specify.

What helps alleviate your hot flashes?

☐ Rest

☐ Working or exercise

☐ Drinking water

☐ Specific foods (please specify)

☐ Change in environment or temperature (please specify)

☐ Herbal formulas, supplements, or vitamins (please specify)

☐ Medications (please specify)

Diagnosing Menopausal-Transition Symptoms

It is reasonable for acupuncturists and Chinese-medicine practitioners to take a holistic approach when treating menopausal-transition
women, making it necessary to observe, diagnose, and treat the accompanying symptoms.

A particularly useful research scale is the Menopause Rating Scale
(MRS), developed by the Berlin Center for Epidemiology and Health
Research. The MRS captures scores for 11 menopausal-transition
symptoms across three subscales.

- Somato-vegetative symptoms: Hot flashes and night sweats,
  sleep problems, heart discomfort, and joint and muscular
  discomfort.

- Psychological symptoms: Depressive mood, irritability, anxiety,
  and physical and mental exhaustion.

- Urogenital symptoms: Sexual problems, bladder problems, and
  vaginal disorders.

The MRS is adequate for customary research. However, its simplistic nature is limiting when it comes to acupuncture and Chinese medicine. As discussed, many patterns of excess and deficiency create the hot-flash environment. It is a multi-layered approach. Research scales are linear in nature and not tailored to capture the details needed in Chinese medicine.

The following menopausal-transition clinical intake not only covers the MRS, but also takes it further by collecting extra details surrounding the symptoms. It provides a detailed look at the patient's hot-flash environment and supports diagnosis.

HEART ISSUES

Rate the following symptom based on the severity: heart discomfort (unusual awareness of heartbeat, heart skipping, heart racing, tightness):

- ☐ None

- ☐ Mild

- ☐ Moderate

- ☐ Severe

- ☐ Extremely severe

Do you experience heart palpitations?   ☐ Yes   ☐ No

Does your heart race?   ☐ Yes   ☐ No

Do you experience heart or chest flutters?   ☐ Yes   ☐ No

Have you been diagnosed with atrial fibrillation?   ☐ Yes   ☐ No

Do you have chest tightness or pain?   ☐ Yes   ☐ No

SLEEP ISSUES

Rate the following symptom based on the severity: sleep problems (difficulty falling asleep, difficulty sleeping through the night, waking up early):

☐ None

☐ Mild

☐ Moderate

☐ Severe

☐ Extremely severe

Are you experiencing any of the following sleep issues?

☐ Difficulty falling asleep

☐ Waking at night

☐ Waking at night to urinate

☐ Difficulty falling back asleep

☐ Waking early

☐ Excessive sleep

Do you feel you get enough sleep?   ☐ Yes   ☐ No

If you do experience these symptoms, when did they begin?

☐ With the onset of menopausal transition

☐ I experienced these symptoms before menopausal transition started

DEPRESSION

Rate the following symptom based on the severity: depressive mood (feeling down, sad, on the verge of tears, lack of drive, mood swings):

☐ None

☐ Mild

☐ Moderate

☐ Severe

☐ Extremely severe

Are you experiencing depression, sadness, or melancholy?   ☐ Yes   ☐ No

If you do experience these symptoms, when did they begin?

☐ With the onset of menopausal transition

☐ I experienced these symptoms before menopausal transition started

IRRITABILITY

Rate the following symptom based on the severity: irritability (feeling nervous, inner tension, feeling aggressive):

☐ None

☐ Mild

☐ Moderate

☐ Severe

☐ Extremely severe

Are you experiencing stress, irritability, tension, anger, or rage?   ☐ Yes   ☐ No

If yes, when did these symptoms begin?

☐ With the onset of menopausal transition

☐ I experienced these symptoms before menopausal transition started

ANXIETY
**Rate the following symptom based on the severity:
anxiety (inner restlessness, feeling panicky):**

☐ None

☐ Mild

☐ Moderate

☐ Severe

☐ Extremely severe

**Are you experiencing anxiety, restlessness,
or panic attacks?**   ☐ Yes ☐ No

If you do experience these symptoms, when did they begin?

☐ With the onset of menopausal transition

☐ I experienced these symptoms before menopausal transition started

ENERGY AND MEMORY
**Rate the following symptom based on the severity: physical
and mental exhaustion (general decrease in performance,
impaired memory, decrease in concentration, forgetfulness):**

☐ None

☐ Mild

☐ Moderate

☐ Severe

☐ Extremely severe

Are you experiencing fatigue?   ☐ Yes   ☐ No

Are you experiencing any of the following cognitive issues?

☐ Impaired memory

☐ Memory loss

☐ Forgetfulness

☐ Poor concentration

☐ Fogginess

If you do experience these symptoms, when did they begin?

☐ With the onset of menopausal transition

☐ I experienced these symptoms before menopausal transition started

SEXUAL PROBLEMS

Rate the following symptom based on the severity: sexual problems (change in sexual desire, change in sexual activity and satisfaction):

☐ None

☐ Mild

☐ Moderate

☐ Severe

☐ Extremely severe

Have you experienced an overall increase in sexual desire?   ☐ Yes   ☐ No

Have you experienced an overall
decrease in sexual desire? ☐ Yes ☐ No

Have you experienced an overall
increase in sexual activity? ☐ Yes ☐ No

Have you experienced an overall
decrease in sexual activity? ☐ Yes ☐ No

Have you experienced an overall
increase in sexual satisfaction? ☐ Yes ☐ No

Have you experienced an overall
decrease in sexual satisfaction? ☐ Yes ☐ No

If do experience these symptoms, when did they begin?

☐ With the onset of menopausal transition

☐ I experienced these symptoms before menopausal transition
started

BLADDER PROBLEMS
Rate the following symptom based on the severity:
bladder problems (difficulty in urinating, increased
need to urinate, bladder incontinence):

☐ None

☐ Mild

☐ Moderate

☐ Severe

☐ Extremely severe

Are you experiencing an increase
with urinary difficulty? ☐ Yes ☐ No

Are you experiencing an increase
in the need to urinate? □ Yes □ No

Are you experiencing an increase
in urination frequency? □ Yes □ No

Are you experiencing urinary incontinence? □ Yes □ No

If you do experience these symptoms, when did they begin?

□ With the onset of menopausal transition

□ I experienced these symptoms before menopausal transition
started

VAGINAL DRYNESS
Rate the following symptom based on the severity:
dryness of vagina (sensation of dryness, burning in
the vagina, difficulty with sexual intercourse):

□ None

□ Mild

□ Moderate

□ Severe

□ Extremely severe

Are you experiencing vaginal dryness? □ Yes □ No

Are you experiencing vaginal burning? □ Yes □ No

Are you experiencing difficulty with
sexual intercourse? □ Yes □ No

Are you experiencing painful
sexual intercourse? □ Yes □ No

If you do experience these symptoms, when did they begin?

☐ With the onset of menopausal transition

☐ I experienced these symptoms before menopausal transition started

JOINT AND MUSCULAR DISCOMFORT

Rate the following symptom based on the severity: joint and muscular discomfort (pain in the joints, rheumatoid complaints):

☐ None

☐ Mild

☐ Moderate

☐ Severe

☐ Extremely severe

Are you experiencing joint or muscular achiness or pain?　　　☐ Yes　☐ No

If you do experience these symptoms, when did they begin?

☐ With the onset of menopausal transition

☐ I experienced these symptoms before menopausal transition started

Tongue and Pulse

The nature of the hot-flash environment, with its excesses and deficiencies, and imbalances of yin and yang, often presents contradictory information. Tongue diagnosis and pulse diagnosis provide the conclusive evidence and reassurance after a detailed hot-flash patient intake.

Theoretically, many patients who need tonifying present with excess fire and are treated with draining techniques. Practitioners may understand hot-flash environment theories and have an indication of the overall pattern, yet may not know for sure what the true condition is or how to best treat the patient.

The tongue and pulse provide hands-on and observational diagnostic answers. Utilized together, the two provide conclusive answers to whether the hot flashes are primarily due to an excess or deficiency environment and where to focus treatment efforts.

Tongue diagnosis confirms the internal environment state. From an auto-mechanic point of view it's like looking beneath the hood at the overall condition of the engine (yin qi aspects). Pulse diagnosis confirms the internal environment function. This is like starting the car to see how well it runs (yang qi aspects). It's cause and effect. The cause is created within the interior and the effect happens throughout the body.

TONGUE

Menopausal-transition patients clinically present with varying degrees of essence depletion, relative yin damage, deficient heat or heat repletion, qi and blood deficiency, qi stagnation, and damp-phlegm accumulation.

Tongue diagnosis allows the practitioner to look directly into the patient's body. Tongue moisture, color, size, and coating reveal the effects of the congenital and acquired constitutions and the current state of the zangfu organs.

A tongue revealing a relative healthy internal environment will present with moisture, and be pale-red, average in size, and have a thin white coating.

Moisture

The lung-spleen-kidney axis provides moisture by generating yuan qi and supplying yin, blood, and body fluids to the tongue.

Many menopausal women will clinically present with a dry tongue. It may even look coarse. A dry tongue supports three ideas: yin and blood internal damage or depletion; presence of internal heat drying out the body fluids; stagnation blocking body fluids from reaching the tongue.

Color

Tongue color provides supporting diagnostic evidence. A red tongue confirms internal heat whether due to repletion, yin deficiency, or stagnation. Deeper shades of red indicate repletion. Redness appearing only along the sides indicates liver heat or fire. A red tongue tip reveals heart fire primarily due to stagnation. A pale tongue confirms general qi and blood deficiency.

Menopausal women commonly present with a pale tongue with enhanced redness along the sides and tip, which confirms a qi and blood deficiency hot-flash environment that is generating a stagnation and heat pattern.

Size

Tongue size reveals congenital and acquired constitution evidence. An emaciated or small tongue indicates relative or absolute or yin and blood depletion. Women can either be born with or develop this over time. Small or emaciated tongues habitually present with a red or crimson color, indicating a long-standing heat pattern, which may derive from relative or absolute or yin and blood depletion.

A swollen tongue indicates excess accumulation due to general qi deficiency with or without stagnation. The kidney, spleen, and lung are in charge of generating qi and promoting body fluids. Qi deficiency cannot engender body fluids and leads to stagnation. Body fluids can no longer circulate, so they accumulate and cause the tongue to swell in size.

Coating

Tongue coating indicates the health of the digestive tract. A thick coating indicates spleen and stomach deficiency with or without stagnation. This is a common clinical presentation, often due to poor or irregular dietary habits. The coating will turn yellow and become drier as digestive stagnation engenders heat and damages yin.

A tongue with little or no coating indicates yin and blood damage or consumption. The coating can disappear from long-standing yangming excess and digestive issues damaging yin, or from relative or absolute zangfu yin deficiency. Tongue cracks are similar in nature.

PULSE

The pulse is the movement of blood through the vessels. The quality of the pulse indicates the current nature of the blood. The current nature of the blood is a direct result of the internal environment, that is the qi and blood, yin and yang, and zangfu organs.

Through the pulse, the doctor can feel how well the internal environment is working. It is like listening to a car when it is idle to see how well it is running. Pulse diagnosis is an art in itself. There are several items of importance to consider when discussing the pulse, including the source of blood, and its circulation, rhythm, and volume.

Blood is a product of the zhen qi, which is generated by the zangfu organs. The overall quality of blood and health of the internal organs is felt in the pulse. A weak pulse or strong pulse indicates the strength of the internal environment.

The blood circulates through the vessels with help from the zangfu organs, primarily the heart and lung. The lung and heart govern qi and blood and are in charge of their movement. When the internal organs are healthy and free from harassment and restriction due to internal disharmony, the blood will circulate freely and the pulse will come and go without effort. Hesitations and restrictions in the pulse are often the result of zangfu organ deficiency and stagnation issues.

The pulse rhythm is affected by the overall yang excitement within the internal environment. Excessive yang qi, heat, and stagnation generate rapid, slippery, and forceful pulses. In contrast, the pulse will be slow, thin, and forceless if the zangfu organs' yang excitement is weak.

Pulse volume is affected by internal excess or deficiency. Excessive patterns generate volume while deficiency patterns diminish volume. Internal excess patterns of heat and stagnation generate full and forceful pulses, whereas thin and forceless pulses are generated from internal deficiency patterns of yin, yang, qi, and blood.

It is quite common to have contradicting excess and deficient pulse rhythm and volume signs, as well as contradicting tongue signs. Case in point: A hot-flash and menopausal-transition patient presents with a small, red tongue with no coating and a large, rapid, forceless pulse. This patient was diagnosed with true yang rising within yin excess due to qi deficiency. With further investigation, the tongue size was congenital in nature, while the color and coating were due to long-standing rising of the true yang. The large pulse was due to yin excess, while the forceless aspect was due to qi deficiency. The rapid nature was due to rising of the true yang within the yin excess. As you can see, diagnosing the hot-flash environment can be challenging at times.

Surgically Induced Hot Flashes

Utter and total disruption of the energetic flows in the body can give rise to erratic symptoms such as those that follow the surgical removal of a woman's uterus and ovaries. After a total hysterectomy and bilateral salpingo-oophorectomy, the vital qi from the uterus and ovaries is dramatically cut off from the brain, heart, and entire body.

This surgery results in surgically induced menopause and has no relation to age or the aging process. It often generates instantaneous hot flashes that are due to the immediate withdrawal of estrogen within the HPO axis.

Having observed and treated many women in the clinical setting with surgical hot flashes, I have found that this type of hot flash is far more difficult to curtail and bring under control. It takes frequent treatments over a longer period of time to recover from the dramatic imbalance created by the surgery.

From the clinical diagnosis point of view, it is necessary to take a closer look at the reasoning behind the necessity to remove the uterus and the ovaries. Often there are substantial menstrual cycle irregularities presenting with severe or constant bleeding. The issue may be a result of internal problems such as cysts, fibroids, uterine prolapse, cancer, pain, endometriosis, etc., resulting in uncontrolled and abnormal bleeding or pain. Over time, the situation may be detrimental to the long-term health or even be life-threatening for the patient.

From a Chinese-medicine standpoint, these derive from various imbalances of the zangfu organs and qi and blood. This can be dysfunction such as qi deficiency being unable to hold the blood within the vessels, stagnation of qi and blood causing irregular bleeding and blood stasis, or heat recklessly forcing blood from the body.

The underlying pattern may be a simple deficiency or stagnation, or it may be complex in nature and composed of excess and deficiency, stagnation, heat, phlegm, and stasis.

The true problem or underlying pattern often remains, even with the immediate surgical removal of the symptom. The true nature of this underlying pattern will become apparent with further discussion about the patient's gynecological health history. Understanding the cause of the problem that required surgery will be the focus of future treatments, in conjunction with quelling the hot flashes.

The primary issue is often contained in the local uterine area or lower jiao. Many women in this particular situation are perfectly healthy otherwise, while other women may have chronic issues, including lifestyle habits that need to be addressed. Whichever the case, surgically induced hot flashes take special care and may require more frequent and consistent treatment to bring them under control.

Many women will go through this procedure well before menopausal transition, sometimes in their thirties or forties. In these cases, there can be another secondary surge of hot flashes around menopausal transition. Practitioners need to make this connection to age and explain to the patient that it's not the previous surgical hot flashes returning, but hot flashes due to menopausal transition.

Pharmaceuticals-Induced Hot Flashes

Certain medications should raise concerns when hot flashes and menopausal-transition patients list them on their intake forms, including thyroid, blood pressure, anxiety, and sleep medications. Recently prescribed drugs suggest that certain symptoms are the direct result of menopausal transition. Long-term prescriptions suggest that the patient has a chronic or complicated pattern that may present a more difficult treatment challenge. The latter does not mean the patient won't respond to acupuncture and herbal medicine; it simply means that the practitioner should make a mental note that it may take longer than normal to curb the hot flashes.

Synthroid (Levothyroxine)

Clinical experience shows that many cases of hot flashes are due to the patient taking this medication.

The clinician must ask the patient if their hot flashes or heat patterns started before or during menopausal transition. Determine how long the patient has been on the medication and if the hot flashes or heat patterns coincide with the start of the medications. Many patients will mention a long history of feeling warm or hot, even before taking the medication.

Synthroid is a thyroid medication. Women are often prescribed this drug because of fatigue or weight gain. When thyroid panels are done, if the numbers are low, the patient is often prescribed Synthroid. In some cases, the symptoms of fatigue go away, while in other cases, they do not.

In Chinese medicine, low thyroid production is due to a history of qi or yang deficiency often going back to childhood. It may be a pre-heaven and/or post-heaven qi issue.

I often mentally red flag cases of hot flashes when the patient is taking Synthroid or other thyroid medications because, clinically, these hot flashes can be more difficult to treat. The theory is that some women may actually require qi or yang boosting herbal formulas, whereas some women may require qi regulation herbal formulas or something else entirely!

The problem with this medication is that it doesn't necessarily act to warm the yang qi; it acts by introducing a heat pathogen into the body. This results in two dueling issues to deal with—treating the underlying condition while concurrently trying to treat and abate the heat side effects of the drug.

Most patients will not entertain the recommendation of reducing and eventually stopping the medication. Many patients have come to rely on it and consider it a necessary treatment.

In my clinical experience, I find that many thyroid issues are treatable with proper lifestyle changes, therapy for emotional issues, necessary vitamin and supplement support, and initial and routine acupuncture and herbal medicine treatments.

Levothyroxine case study: A 48-year-old female patient presented with severe daytime and nighttime hot flashes for several years. Accompanying symptoms included insomnia with frequent waking at night, mental fatigue, physical exhaustion, agitation, and irregular bowel movements. Her pulse was thin and forceless. Her tongue was slightly pale and dry with a red tip.

The original diagnosis was qi stagnation with qi and blood deficiency. I used a general hot-flash excess acupuncture prescription. The patient underwent four acupuncture treatments with little relief. Upon reevaluation, I learned the patient was taking hypothyroid medication, which has the tendency to increase body temperature. Since acupuncture produced little relief from the hot flashes and accompanying symptoms, my conclusion was that the medication was generating the hot flashes.

The patient refused to talk with her doctor about her condition or reducing her dosage. She completed 12 acupuncture treatments with only minor relief. I describe this case to suggest how the acupuncture could have theoretically helped to improve this patient's overall health, making it possible to reduce or cease taking the medication. Also, it is possible that if acupuncture treatments had been started at the onset of the hot flashes, they may have been more successful. I suspect a great deal of stress in this patient's life that may have made it difficult for her to stop her medication.

Tamoxifen

The stomach yangming channel, liver jueyin channel, and chong mai in Chinese medicine dominate the breasts. They are rich in qi and blood but susceptible to qi stagnation and heat.

All tissues in the body, including the breasts, need a healthy supply of nutrition and blood circulation. Tamoxifen is an "anti-estrogen" SERM medication. Tamoxifen blocks estrogen in the body from reaching the breast tissue and is used to help slow the replication of breast-cancer cells.

Chinese medicine sees this type of treatment as disrupting or blocking qi and blood. Tamoxifen works to stop estrogen from feeding breast-cancer cells, but the action of disrupting qi will have an eventual reaction of stagnation and stasis in other areas of the body.

Tamoxifen is absorbed in the intestines and metabolized in the liver, which coincides with the yangming and jueyin channels. Disruption to their physiological functions will lead to qi stagnation, imbalance of yin and yang, and the creation of heat repletion and phlegm.

Based on Chinese medicine, this pharmaceutical has the potential of redirecting the underlying pattern that initially created the breast cancer to another area of the body. Serious side effects of Tamoxifen include a risk of uterine cancer, stroke, and pulmonary embolism. These are all signs of excess qi stagnation generating toxic heat and blood stasis.

Patients often have to take Tamoxifen for five to ten years. Severe, intense, and intractable hot flashes are a common difficult side effect. Clinically, acupuncture can alleviate the hot-flash side effect. Acupuncture is generally most effective if treatment starts near the onset of taking the medication. Routine acupuncture treatment is often necessary to curtail the hot flashes.

Blood-Pressure Medications

Hypertension is an imbalance of yin and yang. It may be an excess of yang qi rising or an issue of yin and blood deficiency generating internal wind. In our profession, it is our objective to control the excess while allowing the deficiency to rebuild. Patients with hypertension are often genetically predisposed to it, while others have it as the result of mismanaged lifestyle habits.

During menopausal transition, the imbalance of yin and yang can cause a disruption in a woman's blood pressure, perhaps increasing systolic blood pressure by >10 points. Diastolic blood pressure is less affected but may increase by >5 points. This is unique to menopausal transition and is common and absolutely normal.

This creates a concern for the Chinese-medicine practitioner. Does the patient require this medication or are they treatable with acupuncture and herbal medicine? Some Western physicians will want to start the patient on medications to bring the blood pressure down to the "normal" 120/80. But is this truly necessary for the patient's overall well-being?

Acupuncture and herbal formulas can provide lasting relief for high blood pressure in some menopausal-transition women. For others, they may only have a limited or temporary relief.

It is clear that for the safety of the patient, drugs are required if the patient's blood pressure is quite high and they are experiencing other hypertension symptoms such as dizziness, headaches, or heart arrhythmias. Even if the blood pressure is only slightly higher than normal, if a woman is experiencing these symptoms during meno-pausal transition, it may warrant the temporary solution of using blood-pressure medications.

Though it is necessary for some women to be on medications to treat the accompanying symptoms of hypertension, when they reach post-menopause and the yin and yang is reestablished, the drugs may no longer be necessary. Patients should be encouraged to explore this possibility with their doctor.

Hypertension case study: A 53-year-old female patient presented with severe hot flashes and night sweating for the previous four to five years. Accompanying symptoms included severe insomnia with waking at night and difficulty falling back asleep, severe mental fatigue, good physical energy, and moderate dizziness. Her pulse was wiry and thin. Her tongue was red along the sides and tip, and puffy and dry.

The original diagnosis was kidney and liver yin deficiency with yang rising. I used a general hot-flash deficiency acupuncture pre-scription. The patient underwent three acupuncture treatments and her hot flashes diminished by 25% but she was still having difficulty sleeping and experiencing dizziness. I added Yintang, PC8, and KI1 calming the spirit and yang anchoring points to the prescription for three additional treatments. The patient's hot flashes dropped by 50%, she was sleeping better, and dizziness was reduced.

This patient received weekly acupuncture treatments for the next 18 weeks. It was found that the patient's symptoms would improve for a short time following treatment and then eventually come back like a seesaw up-down effect. I recommended that the patient saw her primary care physician to check her blood pressure. My hypothesis was that the patient's hot flashes, dizziness, difficulty sleeping, and mental fatigue might be due to a rise in blood pressure when she entered menopausal transition.

The results were conclusive, and the patient did have elevated blood pressure, 140/80. The patient wanted to treat her hypertension with acupuncture and herbal medicine. Again, treatments worked for short durations, but the symptoms always returned. The patient finally decided to take blood-pressure medications, which relieved her symptoms. She now comes in for health-maintenance treatments. The conclusion is that there is a natural tendency for a rise in blood pressure in some women during and after menopausal transition. It is proper to have this discussion with the patient and inform them about medications versus acupuncture and Chinese herbs.

Anxiety Drugs and Sleep Aids

Many underlying hot-flash patterns are the same as those for anxiety and sleep issues. Whether it is yin and yang imbalance, qi and blood deficiency, heat repletion, or stagnations, if you see one of these symptoms in a patient, you are likely to see the others.

Neurotransmitter imbalance (qi dysregulation), nutrient and hormone imbalance (yin and blood deficiency), overactive sympathetic nervous system (yang excess), and adrenal fatigue (qi and essence deficiency) are all common.

A major issue with most anxiety drugs and sleep aids is that patients become dependent on them, both psychologically and physically. First, the drug takes over the physiological process. The natural processes that should manage anxiety and sleep disturbance are not necessary and cease to function as the body becomes accustomed to the "chemical override." Over time, this results in the body being dependent on the drug in order to function naturally. It's like having a servant tie your shoes every day. After a while, when your shoes need tying, you look for the servant instead of tying them yourself.

As with many other drugs, it becomes increasingly more difficult to treat the conditions with acupuncture and herbs and it takes longer to achieve quality results due to the body's dependence on the drugs and the neutralizing effect they have on natural processes in the body. This is an unfortunate but far-too-common scenario in today's clinical setting.

This is regrettable, because the body has amazing capacity for healing. With the natural aid of acupuncture, herbal medicine, vitamins and supplements, and healthy lifestyle changes, the majority of anxiety and insomnia cases could be reversed and eliminated. Even if the drugs are "working" to manage the symptoms, the underlying pattern still exists and will continue to weaken the body.

Conclusion

Too often, patients have a discussion with their doctor about symptoms and are prescribed drugs to treat those symptoms without the essential discussion about if and how they might eventually no longer need the drugs.

Every patient needs to consider whether long-term pharmaceutical treatment is necessary. Are the drugs safe? Are there effective alternatives? Is it possible to taper off the drugs and return their body to a natural state? These are questions that patients should research for themselves and discuss with their doctor.

This discussion holds true for HT. It has established potential risks, and even if it is effective in treating symptoms, it may not be necessary to continue the medications indefinitely. I have found that many physicians are open to considering decreasing and eventually stopping the medications if the patient initiates the discussion.

Many patients are, unfortunately, either psychologically or physically dependent on the prescribed medication and are not ready to make a commitment to change. Some are merely looking for acupuncture and herbal medicine to fix the problem and get rid of the symptom. This is unfortunate, because it prevents them from experiencing the major improvements in their well-being that could be achieved by relatively simple changes in their lifestyles.

The acupuncture and Chinese-medicine profession has many highly skilled and well-trained practitioners. We do work miracles. It is entirely up to the patient and their body to determine if they are ready for the change and the miracle to take place.

Chapter 6

Treating Hot Flashes with Acupuncture

Introduction

Menopausal transition is a time of change and rebirth, and a healing process for the female body. Hot flashes are only a symptom. Heat is the result of a completion of a much larger yinyang cycle and marks the beginning of a new cycle—a rejuvenation!

For this rejuvenation to be successful, yang needs to reignite to replenish depleted yin and refill the body. Estrogen therapy is life support for the old cycle. Prolonged harmful diet and lifestyle habits only drag old problems into the new cycle, making it challenging to recover and start anew.

There are no magic acupuncture points or herbal formulas that treat all hot flashes. There is no single, simple answer to the complex hot-flash environment. Sometimes, the practitioner gets lucky and the first combination works like a charm, but there are many cases where a practitioner must think before finding the right cure.

Clinical work is less about searching for and discovering the secret recipe and more about working diligently every day to find the magic within the individual patient. Repetition develops skills and skills develop into art.

> For the application of the needles it is essential to know how to balance the yin and the yang [qi]. Once yin and yang [qi] are balanced, the essence qi will be luminous… The outstanding practitioner levels the qi. (Unschuld 2016a, p.123)

This quote summarizes an important concept in therapeutic acupuncture. It is particularly apt in directing therapy during menopausal transition. By reestablishing yin and yang balance, women are able to rebloom and their essence becomes luminous.

With the goal of balancing yin and yang, we need to answer a basic diagnostic question: Is the hot flash itself something to clear or something to nourish? A thorough diagnostic process to ascertain the patient's unique hot-flash environment can prevent a lot of wasted time and effort spent simply chasing heat or fire.

It is essential to consider the entire picture. We must analyze the entire zangfu organ system and the organs' relationships with one another. We must investigate the patient's constitution, congenital factors, medical and family history, and gynecological history. We must examine how past and present lifestyle factors are affecting the individual hot-flash environment. The goal is to develop a diagnosis based on the patient's system as a whole and then establish a personalized treatment plan.

Most effective treatment plans for hot-flash patients consist of balancing yin and yang with simultaneous clearing and nourishing treatments utilizing acupuncture, herbs, and lifestyle modifications.

Treatment Approaches to Hot Flashes

Treating hot flashes with acupuncture does not merely revolve around clearing or purging fire from the body. Selecting a few heat clearing points would suffice if this were the case. As we've learned, focus must be on the broader goal of reestablishing a healthy internal environment. By regulating qi and balancing yin and yang, we promote proper generation of qi and blood, allowing fire to be quelled at its source.

A multi-step acupuncture treatment approach needs to be engaged to effectively resolve the hot-flash environment and relieve hot flashes. Any surgeon, architect, or chef will agree that steps need to be established and followed in order to accomplish a set goal. Establishing a successful treatment approach is not difficult. The following steps will provide practitioners with useful information to streamline and improve their clinical efficacy.

Quality Diagnosis

Deeply understanding Chinese-medicine pathophysiology allows for quality diagnosis in the clinical setting. One must understand the cause and development of a particular problem or disease in order to be successful at diagnosing and treating it. By understanding the theories behind hot flashes and how the hot-flash environment is established, we can proactively work to resolve and reestablish balance.

Diagnosis starts immediately when the patient walks through the door. Careful observation can reveal a great deal of information.

Did the patient arrive early or late? Do they seem calm and reserved or boisterous and loud? Are they clothed in many layers or lightly dressed? Is their demeanor lighthearted and joyful, or do they seem irritable, aggressive, or overly scattered? Does the patient show signs of weakness or fatigue, or do they seem energetic? Are they pale or are they full of color?

Patients with heat, stagnation, or excessive yang qi may show up early, are loud, may be wearing lighter than normal clothing, appear vital, and generally have a warm complexion. The qi and blood or yang deficient patients may be late, quiet, dressed warmer than normal, scattered, and weak, and have a pale complexion.

Following the initial observations, the health history, intake questionnaire, and tongue and pulse diagnosis will provide a clearer understanding of and supporting information about the patient's hot-flash environment. Many times, the pattern will be apparent before even asking the first question.

Regulate Qi

Once the diagnosis is confirmed, whether it's an excess or deficient pattern, the primary focus of the initial treatments is on qi regulation. These treatments function much like an oil change for a car—where you first change the fluids and then see how the car runs to see what's wrong with the engine. They work as a diagnostic tool. This initial step is to reestablish proper communication within the zangfu organ system and to promote proper qi and blood circulation along the channels.

The organs need to be able to communicate with each other to generate and build vital qi. The channels need to be open to allow this newly made qi to flow and nourish. Acupuncture stimulation begins the healing process.

The initial treatments also allow the patient to understand acupuncture and the healing process, and give time to develop trust, relax, and let go. Regulating qi clears excess and removes stagnation, which in turn begins the balancing of yin and yang and the promotion and generation of qi and blood. When this system is in place, hot flashes and other menopausal-transition symptoms begin to decrease.

Regulate Digestion

All hot flashes stem from an imbalance within the internal environment. As Li Dong Yuan suggests in the *Pi Wei Lun*, the spleen and stomach are at the center of a healthy system. A poor and weak digestion cannot support a strong and vital system and leads to deficiency of qi and blood and accumulation and stagnation. If the spleen, stomach, and digestive process is not supported and if digestive issues are not addressed, treatments will only have a temporary effect.

Digestive regulation is based on a free and rhythmic movement from top to bottom. The spleen and stomach can function optimally when the complete digestive system is healthy and free of issues. This provides an abundance of qi and blood to the heart and the rest of the zangfu organs, as well as tissues throughout the body. Digestive issues are at the root of many hot-flash situations.

The stomach is at the top of and serves as the beginning of the digestive system. It is prone to excess, stagnation, and fire due to overeating, improper foods, or a lack of support from a deficient spleen. Begin by addressing and subduing any rebellious qi rising from the stomach in the form of acid reflux, belching, hiccups, or nausea.

Continue by regulating qi, nourishing yin, and quelling fire in the stomach. Ask about mouth and tongue sores, bad breath, excessive or incessant hunger, skipping meals, anger or irritability, upper abdominal bloating or pain, or heart palpitations before or after eating. The stomach sits directly below and can easily affect the heart. Hot flashes related to stomach issues can be ameliorated quickly by treating the stomach.

At the center of the digestive process is the spleen. It is common for the spleen to be overworked and suffer from deficiency. This can be more pronounced in the menopausal-transition patient whose body has relied heavily on the spleen to regenerate qi and blood for 30+ years due to the loss during the monthly cycle. Does the patient have no appetite, fatigue, or bloating, or experience frequent gas and intestinal gurgling? It's safe to say that almost every patient can benefit from supporting the spleen. The rebloom of luminous essence, I believe, has much to do with the rejuvenation process of the spleen.

The small and large intestine are situated at the bottom of and complete the final section of the digestion system. As yang fu organs, they are often prone to excess and stagnation due to irregular and improper dietary habits. Over time, the intestines can also become weakened and suffer deficiency that is enhanced by a lack of support from a deficient spleen. Problems within the intestines create bowel-movement disorders including frequency, consistency, and motility issues. Some hot flashes can be traced directly to intestinal and bowel movement problems, especially constipation issues, where repletion builds, rises, and harasses the heart fire. It is important to clear any excesses and tonify the weaknesses.

Constipation case study: A 48-year-old female patient presented with extreme hot flashes and night sweating for the previous eight to ten years. Accompanying symptoms included severe insomnia with waking at night and the inability to fall back asleep, physical and mental fatigue, and a sluggish digestion with constipation. Her pulse was deep and forceful. Her tongue was red and dry with a yellow coating.

The original diagnosis was qi stagnation and liver yin deficiency with deficiency fire. I used a general hot-flash deficiency acupuncture prescription and added KI2. The patient underwent six acupuncture treatments. Her energy levels improved but were not sufficient, her irritability increased, and her hot flashes were only mildly reduced by 20–30%.

Upon reevaluation, I observed the patient had difficulty with constipation with only one bowel movement every three days or so. My hypothesis was that the patient was not responding well because there was qi and heat stagnation in the yangming fueling the hot flashes. I switched the acupuncture focus to promoting digestion. I added SJ6, PC6, RN10, ST28, GB34, LR13, and LU1. After three more acupuncture treatments, the patient was having a bowel movement every day with less difficulty and dryness. The patient's hot flashes dramatically reduced by 80%, her energy increased, and she began sleeping better. My conclusion is that stagnation in the yangming generates heat, which agitates the heart fire while consuming yin.

Treat the Breath

Healthy respiration connects lung and kidney qi and supports the generation and circulation of qi and blood throughout the body. Our system cannot function properly without this connection. Stress and anxiety, as well as lack of activity and poor nourishment, disrupt respiration, disconnect lung and kidney qi communication, and eventually lead to imbalance.

The lung and kidney are susceptible to qi deficiency. Qi stagnation takes advantage of their weakness by blocking and interfering with their communication. Stagnation is slow suffocation. Deficiency and stagnation will generate into one another, and the two are often seen in conjunction.

Stagnation often creates difficulty in expanding the lungs and diaphragm to take deep breaths. This situation is accompanied by shortness of breath, chest tightness or stuffiness, sighing, cough, asthma, or heart palpitations. Qi deficiency causes slower, shallow, and weaker breathing, creating similar symptoms.

The quality and health of the patient's breath is easily observed during the intake and treatment. Watch the patient talk and breathe and look for hesitations and difficulties. Do they breathe into their chest or into their abdomen? Do they hold their breath or talk too much and then have difficulty catching their breath?

Breathing issues must be addressed and treated accordingly to allow proper communication between the lung and kidney. These two organs are the pulse of the zangfu organ system. Much like the digestion, if respiration is not addressed, treatments will only have a temporary or limited effect.

Lung qi stagnation case study: A 61-year-old female patient presented with moderate hot flashes and night sweating for seven years since menopausal transition. Accompanying symptoms included difficulty falling asleep with the need for trazadone, fatigue, brain fog, gas, bloating, constipation, irritability, and anxiety. Her pulse was slippery and rapid. Her tongue was slightly pale and dry with yin cracks.

The original diagnosis was qi stagnation and blood deficiency. I used a general hot flash excess acupuncture prescription and included SJ6. The patient's hot flashes, and other symptoms, improved only slightly after three treatments. Upon reevaluation, I noticed the patient's shallow breathing and inquired about lung issues. The patient had adult onset asthma and used steroids.

It was obvious to me that many of this patient's symptoms were due to qi stagnation in the chest due to lung and kidney qi disconnection. Without the lung qi properly descending, her qi gathered in the chest and was harassing the heart. I also believe habitual and chronic constipation can be the result of the inability of the lung qi to descend. I changed my strategy for the next treatment and switched my focus to descending the lung qi, strengthening the kidney, and harmonizing the liver and spleen. I added LU1, LU6, PC6, and LR13. The patient's hot flashes moderately improved after three more treatments. The patient was breathing better and relying less on her inhaler and sleeping sounder, and anxiety levels decreased. I saw the patient for three more treatments without seeing more improvements. The effectiveness of the acupuncture plateaued for the patient.

I believe this patient could make a full recovery if she was willing to make necessary changes such as incorporating new physical and spiritual activities that would address her breathing habits. The use of asthma steroid inhalers, in my clinical experience, stimulates the lung qi to temporarily descend. The downside is they dry out the lung yin, further weakening the lung qi. Without breaking this cycle, it is difficult to see lasting effects.

Treat the Deficiency

It is safe and easy to add points to support deficiency from the very beginning. It is often necessary to do so in order for mechanisms to work properly. You cannot properly and continually move qi without a source of new qi.

Targeting deficiencies of qi, blood, yin, yang, and essence becomes easier once the qi, digestion, and respiration begin to regulate from the initial treatments. Sometimes it is not as necessary to tonify, because once the engine is running properly, the regeneration process of qi and blood is underway.

Treat the Heat

Targeting heat directly is only necessary after the above procedures have been established. Adding points to address heat or fire from the beginning is normal and safe, but keep heat clearing to a minimum at the beginning. Focusing along one or two channels is sufficient in most cases.

However, if heat and fire signs are not resolving at a natural pace along with treatments, it is time to add points to directly address the heat. Keep in mind that many hot-flash cases will not begin abating until after treatments are well underway. Practitioners cannot rush this process and need to practice patience.

Treat the Shen

Our shen or spirit requires continual support from a harmonious and robust zangfu organ system. Imbalances of heat, stagnation, and deficiency increase around menopausal transition, allowing for an increase in spirit problems such as mental and physical fatigue, sleep issues, poor concentration, anxiety, and depression.

By and large, low-grade tendencies of this nature are normal around menopausal transition. If mild in nature, they tend to naturally decline or disappear over time and are easily controlled with acupuncture treatments. If heightened shen issues continue after treatments have been established, it becomes necessary to add points to address the problems. Even if hot flashes are the primary reason for treatments, it is quite easy to make necessary adjustments to treat shen disturbances.

Some patients will have a history of emotional imbalances. It is essential to identify any history of emotional issues and medications during the intake process. Patients in this category may have heightened problems with anxiety, depression, melancholy, resentment, or agitation, and treatments may need to be adjusted to address these underlying issues.

Ministerial fire case study: A 57-year-old female patient presented with moderate to severe hot flashes and night sweating. Her hot flashes increased in intensity at night but the patient was always hot. Accompanying symptoms included a myriad of physical pains and fibromyalgia stemming from chronic joint and muscle conditions, adult-onset asthma, dry eyes, chronic sinus issues, teeth grinding, skin itchiness, heartburn, constipation, pelvic floor weakness, urinary incontinence, and hypertension. The patient slept well, and was jovial, but seemed shen disturbed because she avoided certain questions and kept to her narrative. She liked to exercise "occasionally" but could not lose weight. She was only 20 pounds overweight but looked plump, as if there were pressure from the inside out. Her complexion was pale, pulse was forceful and slippery, and tongue was pale purple, puffy, and dry.

The original diagnosis was stirring of ministerial fire due to lung and spleen qi deficiency and kidney essence deficiency. The patient was somewhat sensitive to needle insertion and qi sensations. Nourishing points mildly agitated symptoms, while clearing and draining points left the patient fatigued. Utilizing a qi and phlegm resolving and calming the spirit acupuncture prescription (DU20, DU24, Yintang, RN14, RN6, RN4, LR13, PC6, LI11, SJ6, SP9, GB34, LR3, KI3) produced the best results.

She underwent 30 acupuncture treatments over the course

of three years, with limited success. Her progress was hindered as she was infrequent with her treatment schedule, which did not foster continual progress. In the clinical setting, women who fall into this category often have a complex set of contradicting symptoms that makes diagnosis and treatment difficult. I suspect that in some cases there are unresolved emotional issues and perhaps a history of mental, emotional, or physical abuse.

Treat Chronic Damp-Phlegm

Damp-phlegm patterns are often chronic in nature and are due to complex and long-standing excess deficiency scenarios. It is said that all chronic conditions are the result of phlegm. Addressing and directly treating dampness and phlegm may be required when hot flashes and menopausal-transition symptoms are resistant to treatments. To effectively resolve chronic damp-phlegm conditions, it is often necessary for patients to make changes to their lifestyle habits, addressing diet, activity, and stress.

Acupuncture Hypersensitivity and Needling Techniques

Menopausal-transition patients in general respond quite well to acupuncture treatments and enjoy the relaxation effects. A patient once said that she felt guilty because she felt so good afterwards. In contrast, I've also had patients terminate treatment because they didn't enjoy the acupuncture.

Over the years, I've seen a tendency for patients to either love or dislike acupuncture treatments. I began taking notes on how well each patient responded to treatments. I questioned patients about what they liked and disliked about their acupuncture treatments. Patients often responded with compliments, saying they felt better, happier, and healthier. On the negative side, patient dislikes predominantly revolved around needle pain or sensitivity and the inability to relax.

There is a natural increase in anxiety levels in today's society. It's also common to see an increase in anxiety when women enter menopausal transition. Women have much to deal with, including stress around finances, career, family, relationships, and social responsibilities. Some have better luck balancing life than others. It is completely natural for some patients to respond better to acupuncture than other patients.

The healing process begins when the nervous system is able to switch back into a parasympathetic state. The body repairs itself a little more each time the patient relaxes while receiving treatment.

In order to help anxious patients who cannot relax, it is essential to tailor treatments in a way that means they can enjoy treatments and feel better. By acknowledging that some patients weren't responding favorably and changing some key clinical understandings and treatment approaches, I have been able to help more patients. These changes increased my overall clinical efficacy in treating hot flashes and menopausal-transition patients.

Acupuncture Hypersensitivity

Clinically, there is a noticeable increase in needle sensitivity in menopausal-transition women, and many hot-flash patients are more sensitive to acupuncture.

Acupuncture is a stimulus that activates the body's healing potential. When the needle is inserted correctly, it stimulates this healing response called "deqi" or the arrival of qi. The arrival of qi is necessary, and it activates sensations of warmth, twinges, distension, heaviness, tingling, or numbness, all of which are minor, tolerable, and temporary. Afterwards, these sensations fade and the patient is able to relax and enjoy their healing journey. Every patient has needle sensitivity to some extent, even if it is very minor. It can become problematic when a patient's sensitivity is higher than normal.

Needle sensitivity in itself is not a medical problem. Some patients' nervous systems are simply hyperstimulable and hypersensitive. This may actually be clinically beneficial for some, where the healing response is quickly achieved. Some patients in this category are upset or ashamed because they really want to relax and heal. It is up to the practitioner to reassure them that needle sensitivity is a natural occurrence.

Administering effective and gentle treatments for patients in this category presents its challenges. Needle sensitivity in Chinese medicine is due to many factors, including the patient's natural constitution, quality of qi and blood, balance and strength of yin and yang, stagnation issues, and heat factors. Keep in mind that this is a generalization and does not mean that every patient with a specific pattern or constitution will or will not be hypersensitive to acupuncture.

Excess and Deficiency

Excess and deficiency patterns play a primary role in acupuncture sensitivity. The acupuncture needle achieves a qi response when the qi is stronger and more active, which is true in excess patterns. Stagnation, repletion, and excessive yang qi patterns carry a greater chance at having a strong deqi or qi sensation response and equal an increase in needle sensitivity potential. Deficiency patterns are more apt to have a weaker deqi or qi sensation response and a decreased needle sensitivity potential. There are exceptions where yin excess may have a decreased potential, while yin or blood deficiency may have an increased potential.

Qi and Blood

The quality of qi and blood factor into patient acupuncture sensitivity and how well they are able to relax on the treatment table. Generalized qi and blood deficient patients are typically ready to enjoy their time to relax or sleep during treatments and are, not surprisingly, easy to treat. Their bodies are receptive to the needles, almost craving the stimulation.

Qi deficiency patients tend to be less sensitive to the needles. There are really no issues as long as the practitioner's acupuncture techniques and point location are fine.

Even if the qi is weak, an increase in needle sensitivity may arise in patients with pronounced blood deficiency. The potential for this increase is because the tissues are undernourished and dry, causing the nerves to be hypersensitive. Blood deficiency often equates to increased anxiety.

Yin and Yang

The balance of yin and yang strength perhaps best illustrates and plays the largest role in patient acupuncture sensitivity. Patients with exuberant yang qi can be quite anxious and hypersensitive to acupuncture. When yang qi is strong, it becomes active and stimulable. The act of inserting a needle into this body is like holding a metal rod up towards the sky in a lightning storm.

Once a patient's qi becomes overactivated, it triggers a nervous response that reverberates throughout the body. Once this begins, it becomes increasingly difficult to continue needling without generating more sensitivity, much like hitting a gong over and over again. When finding oneself in this situation, it is best to allow the patient's system to calm down. It may be necessary to withdraw the sensitive needles, change needle gauge, and choose an alternative and less-sensitive point prescription.

Yin deficiency is similar to blood deficiency. The patient's tissues are undernourished and there is less yin flowing through the tissues and channels. The acupuncture sensitivity potential is heightened due to the unopposed yang qi, thus allowing for a hyperactive nervous system.

Stagnation

Stagnation consists of qi, blood, and body fluids and can take place anywhere within the zangfu organs or along the channel system. Patients with stagnation can be very sensitive to acupuncture, depending on the underlying cause.

It is easy to observe heightened clinical needle sensitivity as a result of sustained stress, fatigue, lack of sleep, diet, and other lifestyle habits that amplify and strain the sympathetic nervous system. Successful needle administration will have a great effect on these patients by calming down and returning the system back to a parasympathetic state. Stagnation patients need this break in the cycle to unwind and to allow the healing response to take place.

Qi stagnation hot-flash case study: A 59-year-old female patient presented with moderate and chronic daytime and nighttime hot flashes. The patient experienced a normal menopausal transition. She suffered from high stress both at work and when taking care of her elderly parents. She had a history of allergies and itchy and weeping skin sores presenting mainly on the extremities and occasionally on the chest and face that were triggered by stress and dietary choices. In general, she had good energy and digestion. Her pulse was deep and forceful. Her tongue was slightly purple and dry with a red tip.

I originally diagnosed this patient with qi stagnation and damp-heat accumulation.

I used a general hot-flash excess acupuncture prescription. After a series of four treatments, the patient's daytime and night-time hot flashes subsided by 75%. The patient's skin improved and she had more energy.

Many hot flashes are exacerbated by chronic qi stagnation due to high stress. When the liver qi is soothed, dampness is drained, the spleen recovers, and fire is abated. I have treated this patient off and on for several years. She usually comes in for two to three maintenance treatments one or two times per year. Her stress levels rarely change and she always seems frustrated. She always improves with acupuncture, relaxation, and taking vacations, and often takes herbal formulas such as Jia Wei Xiao Yao San and skin-related formulas.

Needling Techniques

Every practitioner will inevitably experience a patient with acupuncture hypersensitivity. These patients will respond better to acupuncture and their bodies will be more receptive to the treatment when the practitioner modifies a number of treatment methods.

Adapted clinical skills and treatment styles include changing needle brands, selecting an appropriate needle gauge and length, altering point prescriptions and the insertion sequence, using fewer needles, improving needling techniques, adjusting the length of treatment, and determining the best time of day for treatment. Consider these issues and modifications and experiment to reduce needle sensitivity.

Hypersensitivity is usually worse at the initiation of treatment. It diminishes over time as the body improves through the healing process.

Types of Needles

The quality of acupuncture needle is the first factor to consider. Get rid of the inexpensive needles. Low-cost brands equal lower quality. The tips are inferior to those of the well-known brands. High-quality needles have sharper tips that allow for a cleaner and less painful puncture when piercing the skin. The needle will speak for itself.

Needle gauge may also be an issue. In most instances, 34-gauge is appropriate. Anything thicker is not warranted for treating hot flashes. Lower-gauge needles are appropriate for longer needles where the practitioner needs to insert and treat deeper into the body, such as for large abdomens and hip issues.

Patients are more susceptible to acupuncture hypersensitivity in areas with less fat tissue and tighter skin, and along nerve innervations. Common areas include the ankles, wrists, hands, and feet. The abdomen may also be a particularly sensitive area in lean patients. In these cases, if the patient is still prone to sensitivity, changing to a 36- or 38-gauge needle is appropriate.

Needle-Insertion Techniques

Sometimes the problem is not the needle, but the practitioner's skills in point location and insertion technique. Correctly locating each acupuncture point is key, not only to obtain the best healing response, but also to lessen unwarranted patient discomfort. Even seasoned acupuncturists have less-than-perfect point-location skills. If one repeatedly elicits discomfort at one or multiple acupuncture points, it is best to recheck the location and examine the insertion techniques.

Acupuncture points have a specified depth where correct deqi can be activated. It is just like drilling a well to find water: too shallow or too deep will not bring fresh water. Acupuncture follows the same principles. The depth of insertion is a crucial factor in patient comfort.

For example, there's greater potential for increased sensitivity and discomfort when the needle is caught cross grain in the tissues or stuck in the superficial cutaneous tissues after insertion. No matter what gauge the needle is, there is greater sensitivity in the shallow layers of the body due to the vast network of cutaneous nerves. On the other hand, deep insertions may also elicit sensitivity, pain, or discomfort. The deeper regions contain larger vessels and nerves. When stimulated, there is a potential for large and surprising jolts of aches, electrical discomfort, and pain.

Point Prescription and Sequence

It is sometimes necessary to change acupuncture-point prescriptions because of hypersensitivity. It's a trap to think there is only one point or one particular point formula that will help cure the patient. There is always an alternative point and point prescription that will produce a similar effect.

It is also beneficial to needle less-sensitive points first. Certain points are easier to needle and carry less risk of overstimulation. Start with them before moving on to more sensitive points. In general, points on the torso and in the larger muscles are less sensitive. For example, when treating a hypersensitive patient, it may be beneficial to needle abdominal points first and LI4 later.

Every body is unique. Blood vessels and nerves may not have the exact trajectory or depth from one person to the next. Correct point location avoids problematic areas, but from time to time, certain points will be an issue because a nerve is too shallow and hyperstimulable or a blood vessel is following a slightly different innervation.

Make a note of acupuncture points that are challenging for each patient. Switch to less sensitive points along the same channel if necessary, such as needling SP9 over SP6. Avoid consistent problematic points. Less is more with sensitive patients.

Don't be afraid to change points. After all, the essence of the healing process resides in the patient's ability to relax and feel comfortable. Utilizing fewer points and points that are less sensitive will yield greater results in the long term.

Length of Treatment

Patients respond differently to the overall length of individual treatment sessions. Some prefer long treatments while others are perfectly fine with a shorter time. The average length of time for the healing response to be activated and achieved is 20–25 minutes. This time frame is usually adequate for most excess patterns. For deficient patterns, 30–35 minutes or longer is sufficient. Sedation is faster than stimulation.

It is easy to tell what the patient's body requires after a few treatments. Check in with your patients to determine whether they are able to relax. Some will fall asleep while others will lay there watching the clock. It's important to talk with your patient and ask them how much time they prefer. Some will want to go for as long as you will allow them.

Energetic and hypersensitive patients will let you know they are fine with less time. Over the course of several treatments, stagnation and repletion subsides and nervous systems become easier to regulate. Patients will begin to tap into their inner resources and deepen relaxation. They will naturally want to stay for longer treatments.

In extreme cases, some women cannot lay still for any significant amount of time. Patients in this situation continually ask if they are done or how much longer they have left. This type of patient is challenging to treat and may not be suited to acupuncture. The practitioner may need to prescribe herbal formulas and utilize other types of therapies such as auricular seed therapy, laser therapy, moxibustion, and tuina, to calm the patient's nervous system to activate the healing response.

Time of Day

Treatment time of day plays a role in acupuncture hypersensitivity. Menopausal transition is composed of excess and deficiency patterns. Hot-flash patients can be more sensitive in the morning, afternoon, or evening based on their overall hot-flash environment.

Our vital qi is robust when we awake and is gradually depleted over the course of the day. Daybreak to noontime is yang in nature. Increased qi exists and hot flashes can be excessive. Conversely, afternoon to midnight is yin in nature. Depleted qi exists and hot flashes can rise to the surface.

Applying this principle, a deficient patient may be relaxed and able to obtain a positive healing response during a morning treatment when their vital qi is abundant from being restored overnight. However, as their qi is depleted over the course of a day, this same patient becomes more acupuncture sensitive in the evening.

An excess patient may respond in the opposite manner. They may have increased sensitivity in the morning because their qi is overly abundant. As their qi becomes more stable throughout the day, they may be able to obtain a positive healing response in the evening.

A further complication exists because these two scenarios can be reversed. Excess patients may be increasingly sensitive in the evening when qi is depleted and there is unabated yang qi. Deficient patients may be increasingly sensitive in the morning because they have not built up an adequate supply of vital qi overnight, allowing for increased morning yang qi.

It is interesting to observe these differences in the clinic. In certain circumstances, it may be necessary to administer treatment at another time of day to determine if the acupuncture sensitivity changes.

Traditional Hot-Flash Acupuncture Prescriptions

Menopausal-transition acupuncture prescriptions can be found in multiple acupuncture and Chinese-medicine source texts. Hot-flash acupuncture prescriptions, on the other hand, are rather limited. Theoretically, utilizing prescriptions targeting menopausal-transition Chinese-medicine patterns can treat hot flashes.

Practitioners face a challenge. Hot flashes and menopausal-transition acupuncture prescriptions are not congruent from one source to the next. Authors, scholars, and practitioners alike share their personal knowledge, experience, and understanding of acupuncture and Chinese medicine based on the classical sources and theories they were taught. Common menopausal-transition acupuncture styles revolve around traditional zangfu theory, five-phase theory, and eight-confluent-point theory.

It would be ideal for the medical community at large if every Chinese-medicine lineage were traced back to one original source of reference, but this is not the case. In fact, there are so many styles and branches of acupuncture and Chinese medicine, it is nearly impossible to know, let alone practice, them all well.

Practicing one particular branch or style of Chinese medicine well and gaining mastery takes a lifetime. No one can say that one particular branch or style is better overall than the other. What matters most is how well the specific knowledge translates to and how effective it is in the clinical setting.

Tidal Heat Effusion: Acupuncture Prescriptions

A good foundational chao re source comes from *A Practical Dictionary of Chinese Medicine* (Wiseman and Ye 1998, p.613) and covers tidal heat effusion patterns along with definitions of times of day tidal heat effusion arises, accompanying symptoms, and proposed acupuncture prescriptions.

YIN AND BLOOD DEFICIENCY

Yin deficiency and blood depletion tidal heat effusion generally manifests during the afternoon, evening, or night. Accompanying symptoms include waves of low-grade heat that come and go, heat in the palms and soles, heart vexation, insomnia, heart palpitations, night sweating, a red tongue with little coating, and a fine and rapid pulse. This type is most closely related to hot flashes during menopausal transition.

The base acupuncture formula for yin deficiency and blood depletion is: KI2 (Rangu) 然谷, KI6 (Zhaohai) 照海, SP6 (Sanyinjiao) 三阴交, HT8 (Shaofu) 少府, HT7 (Shenmen) 神门, LU10 (Yuji) 鱼际, DU14 (Dazhui) 大椎, PC5 (Jianshi) 间使.

I find two parts of this prescription are particularly beneficial in the clinic: The first is the use of two points along a single meridian or channel, like KI2 and KI6. I find this to be a useful technique clinically, especially along the kidney and spleen channel.

The second is the use of KI2 and HT8. Both are ying-spring points on the dueling shaoyin channels. I find both points useful specifically for directly quelling hot flashes. I believe these two points are able to clear heart fire within the shaoyin and return water fire balance back to the kidney and heart. These two points can be added to any hot-flash prescription for this reason.

YANGMING EXCESS

Yangming excess tidal heat effusion is different than the others because it is a constant heat effusion. It is also known as "late-afternoon tidal heat effusion" because the heat becomes increasingly more pronounced at 3–5pm. Accompanying symptoms include streaming sweat on the hands and feet, fullness and pain in the abdomen, constipation, vexation and agitation, a dry and yellow tongue coating, and a deep and forceful pulse.

The base acupuncture formula for yangming excess is: ST44 (Neiting) 内庭, LI4 (Hegu) 合谷, LI11 (Quchi) 曲池, LI6 (Pianli) 偏历, ST36 (Zusanli) 足三里, BL25 (Dachangshu) 大肠俞, DU14 (Dazhui) 大椎, PC5 (Jianshi) 间使.

This prescription is purely for opening and clearing heat from the yangming channels. It is effective for treating excess and instances of febrile disease. Some of the listed points can be utilized for quelling hot flashes in patients with heat repletion or stagnation conditions.

SPLEEN AND STOMACH QI DEFICIENCY

Spleen and stomach qi deficiency tidal heat effusion causes morning heat effusion and then abates. Accompanying symptoms include lassitude, weakness of the limbs, spontaneous sweating, a white complexion, a pale tongue, and a fine or weak pulse.

The base acupuncture formula for Spleen and Stomach Qi Deficiency is: BL20 (Pishu) 脾俞, BL21 (Weishu) 胃俞, RN6 (Qihai) 气海, RN12 (Zhongwan) 中脘, ST36 (Zusanli) 足三里, DU14 (Dazhui) 大椎.

Spleen and stomach qi deficiency is a common root problem in hot-flash environments. RN6 and ST36 can easily be adopted into any deficiency prescription. These acupoints are not warranted and may aggravate the situation if the patient has heat repletion or signs of stagnation.

DAMP-EVIL OBSTRUCTION

Damp-evil obstruction tidal heat effusion is due to the external attack of summer-heat. The hot and humid weather of late-summer penetrates and enters the body, impairing the spleen and stomach qi. This form of tidal heat effusion has a gradual recovery with the arrival of autumn. Accompanying symptoms include low-grade fever, thirst, loss of appetite, vexation, agitation, fatigue, weakness, diarrhea, a greasy tongue coating, and a fine and rapid pulse.

The base acupuncture formula for damp-evil obstruction is: PC6 (Neiguan) 内关, LI4 (Hegu) 合谷, ST36 (Zusanli) 足三里, DU14 (Dazhui) 大椎, RN6 (Qihai) 气海, BL20 (Pishu) 脾俞.

Damp-evil obstruction is traditionally due to weather-related issues but can also be the result of food-related issues such as spoiled or contaminated food or water, or in situations where the food is too rich and heavy for the patient's digestion. Patients with a history of traveling to other countries or who have dietary irregularities may present with this pattern in the clinic. Although this prescription is ideal for weather-related issues, it may not be a complete formula for treating food-related issues.

BLOOD STASIS

Blood stasis tidal heat effusion is due to long-standing static blood depression within the body. Stasis gives rise to chronic afternoon tidal heat effusion. Accompanying symptoms include a dry mouth and throat, pain in the body, a blue or purplish tongue with possible macules, and a rough and fine pulse.

The base acupuncture formula for blood stasis is: BL17 (Geshu) 膈俞, SP10 (Xuehai) 血海, LI4 (Hegu) 合谷, LR3 (Taichong) 太冲, SP6 (Sanyinjiao) 三阴交, KI6 (Zhaohai) 照海, KI2 (Rangu) 然谷, LR2 (Xingjian) 行间.

The four gates (LI4 and LR3) along with SP6 are effective additions for regulating qi and blood in most hot-flash environments, whether excess or deficient.

Menopause—Patterns and Acupuncture Prescriptions

A well-rounded and complete source for menopausal-transition acupuncture prescriptions comes from the *Modern Acupuncture and Moxibustion Treatment Success Compendium* 现代针灸治疗大成 (Wu, Zhang, and Jin 2006) published by the Chinese Medicine Science and Technology Publishing Society. It is worth noting that menopause is listed among the neurological disorders and not gynecological disorders in this compendium. Below are several modern acupuncture prescriptions, along with a commentary.

The first sets of acupuncture-point prescriptions are fairly standardized for their set zangfu organ pattern. Each one could theoretically be used to treat almost any clinical patient, not just menopausal-transition patients. Hot-flash environments often consist of more than one pattern, making these prescriptions interchangeable as clinically needed.

- Kidney yin deficiency: KI3 (Taixi) 太溪, SP6 (Sanyinjiao) 三阴交, KI7 (Fuliu) 复溜, BL23 (Shenshu) 肾俞.

- Kidney yang deficiency: RN4 (Guanyuan) 关元, DU4 (Mingmen) 命门, BL23 (Shenshu) 肾俞, ST36 (Zusanli) 足三里.

- Heart and spleen qi deficiency: HT7 (Shenmen) 神门, PC6 (Neiguan) 内关, SP6 (Sanyinjiao) 三阴交, ST36 (Zusanli) 足三里, BL15 (Xinshu) 心俞, BL20 (Pishu) 脾俞.

- Central qi (zhong qi) of the spleen and stomach deficiency: DU20 (Baihui) 百会, RN4 (Guanyuan) 关元, ST36 (Zusanli) 足三里, RN12 (Zhongwan) 中脘, RN6 (Qihai) 气海, BL20 (Pishu) 脾俞.

- Liver depression with blood stasis and qi stagnation: LR3 (Taichong) 太冲, LI11 (Quchi) 曲池, SP10 (Xuehai) 血海, LR2 (Xingjian) 行间, BL17 (Geshu) 膈俞, PC7 (Daling) 大陵, SP6 (Sanyinjiao) 三阴交, LI4 (Hegu) 合谷, BL32 (Ciliao) 次髎.

- Damp-phlegm stagnation: Yintang (M-HN-3) 印堂, DU20 (Baihui) 百会, RN12 (Zhongwan) 中脘, ST40 (Fenglong) 丰隆, SP10 (Xuehai) 血海, SP6 (Sanyinjiao) 三阴交, BL17 (Geshu) 膈俞, GB20 (Fengchi) 风池.

- Blood deficiency with blood stasis: BL20 (Pishu) 脾俞, BL23 (Shenshu) 肾俞, ST36 (Zusanli) 足三里, RN4 (Guanyuan) 关元, SP10 (Xuehai) 血海, SP6 (Sanyinjiao) 三阴交, SP1 (Yinbai) 隐白, SP9 (Yinlingquan) 阴陵泉. (Wu, Zhang, and Jin 2006, pp.1030–1031)

COMMENTARY

Even though they seem straightforward, there are some interesting concepts embedded in these acupuncture-point prescriptions. When reviewing menopausal-transition pathophysiology, focus revolves not only around kidney deficiency, but equally around the spleen. This is because the spleen is in charge of qi and blood production, which needs continuous replenishment throughout life, and especially during menopausal transition. This theory is supported, as SP6, BL20, and a few kidney points are utilized in almost every prescription. It is noteworthy that KI6 and HT6, which are considered by some to be indispensable points for treating hot flashes, are not included in any of these prescriptions.

Menopausal transition includes hot flashes and many shen-related symptoms such as insomnia and anxiety. It is also noteworthy that very few calming the spirit points, including HT7, are included. Neither are heat clearing points, including ying-spring points. This supports the concept that clearing heat or calming shen may not be a priority or necessary, and hot flashes and other somatic issues will naturally resolve once the qi and blood are supported.

Clinical Research

In 2008, I completed research observing the clinical effects of acupuncture on treating perimenopausal symptoms and improving understanding of the mechanisms behind the effects. As a new doctor, I made several rookie mistakes through the course of my clinical-research process. Considering mistakes I made in research protocols, the research is, in itself, scientifically invalid.

It was, of course, disappointing to find my research was flawed. In hindsight, though, I find my efforts served two important purposes. I did demonstrate clinically how well a set of acupuncture points can be used to treat menopausal-transition symptoms. More importantly, discoveries and new theories that materialized during the research fueled the next 12 years of personal clinical investigations into hot flashes and served as a foundation and starting point for this book.

Research Methods

Forty-two women applied to participate in the study. After a detailed initial intake, 11 women were excused for not meeting the requirements. The 31 remaining women were able to participate in the study. Of these, six women were disqualified for not completing the research. There were 25 women who met all of the qualifications and specifications and finished the 12-week research study. The main threats inferring with data in this type of investigative research are that there is no control group and it is not a blinded study.

INCLUSION CRITERIA
Women had to be age 35–65 and to present with common menopausal-transition symptoms including hot flashes, night sweats, sleep irregularities, heart discomfort or palpitations, anxiety, melancholy or depression, heavy or prolonged menses, irregular or ceasing of menses, vaginal irregularities, sexual problems, bladder irregularities, fatigue and weakness, and arthralgia. An essential requirement was that symptoms must have started gradually during the time of menopausal transition, around the age of 45–55 years old. Participating women needed to commit to one acupuncture treatment per week for a 12-week treatment course.

EXCLUSION CRITERIA
Women were excluded if they did not meet the inclusion criteria or if there was insufficient evidence that their symptoms were a direct result of menopausal transition.

PRIMARY OBSERVATION INSTRUMENT
The primary instrument and index adopted was the Menopause Rating Scale (MRS), developed by the Berlin Center for Epidemiology and

Health Research. Each subject completed the MRS at the beginning and end of the study. All scores were tallied and the difference between the beginning and finished scores were evaluated.

The MRS is a self-administrable patient questionnaire. It measures 11 symptoms in three categories: somato-vegetative symptoms; psychological symptoms; urogenital symptoms. One downfall of using this style of scale is that it only measures patient severity of subjectively perceived complaints.

TREATMENT METHODS

Creating an acupuncture-point prescription for the research posed challenges. The goal was to identify a standardized selection of acupuncture points to treat all of the symptoms of menopausal transition rather than designing individualized point prescriptions based on Chinese-medicine pattern differentiation for each subject.

All of the acupuncture points and prescriptions used in well over 100 menopause Chinese research studies and articles were cataloged. With analysis, common patterns were identified. Some acupoints were used far more often than others. From these patterns, a core group of selected acupuncture points was chosen to be used with the subjects in the research.

The hope was that the study would be successful and the identified acupuncture-point prescription could be applied by all practitioners of Chinese and Western medicine to treat menopausal-transition symptoms without having to utilize Chinese-medicine pattern differentiation.

All acupoints selected were located on the anterior portion of the body. This allowed for an easy supine positional treatment, eliminating the need to insert needles on both the front and back of the body. This was efficient, although including back-shu points as listed in many acupuncture textbooks may have increased therapeutic effectiveness.

The idea behind this study was to make the treatment simple, fast, and effective. The acupuncture prescription developed was: DU20 (Baihui) 百会, HT7 (Shenmen) 神门, PC6 (Neiguan) 内关, LI4 (Hegu) 合谷, RN6 (Qihai) 气海, RN4 (Guanyuan) 关元, ST36 (Zusanli) 足三里, SP6 (Sanyinjiao) 三阴交, KI3 (Taixi) 太溪, LR3 (Taichong) 太冲. This set of points is the targeted primary focus of treatment during menopausal transition, chiefly tonifying and nourishing the kidney essence and yin and boosting the yang while harmonizing the functions of the heart, liver, and spleen.

Auricular seed therapy was added to help maintain the effects of the treatment over the course of one week until the next treatment. The auricular acupuncture prescription used was: Shenmen 神门, Uterus 子宫, Kidney 肾, Heart 心, Liver 肝, Spleen 脾, Pituitary 脑垂体, Sympathetic 交感, Endocrine 内分泌, Neurasthenia 神经衰弱点.

Treatment was administered once per week for 12 weeks. The acupuncture needles were retained for 20 minutes during each treatment. After the body acupuncture, seed acupuncture therapy was applied and kept in place for three to five days. Participants were instructed to press the seeds to induce sensation several times per day. The seeds were applied to one ear, alternating ears with each treatment, to maintain fresh stimulation of the auricular points.

Study Results

Sample reporting was based and scored using the MRS.

All 25 participants with somato-vegetative symptoms reported decreased overall severity: 81% for those with hot flashes, 74% for those with heart discomfort, 92% for those with sleep problems, and 95% for those with joint and muscular discomfort.

All but one (24 of 25, 96%) of the participants with psychological symptoms reported decreased overall severity: 87% of the 23 with depressive mood, 78% of the 23 with irritability, 89% of the 19 with anxiety, and 92% of the 25 with physical and mental exhaustion at baseline.

In total, 20 of 22 participants (91%) with urogenital symptoms reported decreased overall severity: 89% of the 19 with sexual problems, 100% of the 17 with bladder problems, and 86% of the 14 with dryness of the vagina.

One participant reported an increase in sexual problems from mild to moderate. Five participants reported onset of a symptom during the treatment period, one each for: depressive mood, sexual problems, anxiety, bladder problems, or joint and muscular discomfort.

Somato-Vegetative Symptoms: Results and Clinical Observations

HOT FLASHES AND NIGHT SWEATS

Hot flashes and night sweats are common manifestations seen in menopausal-transition women and were the chief complaints for most women in the study. Acupuncture treatments reduced intensity, frequency, and duration for most women at a gradual rate. Few women experienced fast relief after two to three treatments. There was a noticeable shift after five to six treatments. Intensity, frequency, and duration were all relieved at an equal rate.

Night sweats were relieved at the same rate as hot flashes. There was a 59% overall reduction in hot flashes and night sweating manifestations by the end of the study.

From the results, it can be deduced that acupuncture can effectively relieve hot flashes for many patients when they are due to natural aging effects. However, it should be noted that when hot flashes are surgically or pharmaceutically generated, or complicated by medications, long-term drug use, or chronic illness, the use of Chinese herbal medicine in conjunction with acupuncture is suggested.

SLEEP PROBLEMS

Sleep disorders including trouble falling asleep, trouble staying asleep, frequent waking at night, and waking early in the morning are multifaceted in nature. All sleep problems are categorized as insomnia in Chinese medicine.

Acupuncture treatments had a positive effect on the subjects' sleep patterns. In most cases, women reported being able to fall asleep much more easily and without any complaints by the end of the study. Perhaps more noteworthy was improvement in the symptom of waking in the middle of the night reported by many women in the study. Observation over the three-month study showed a slow, gradual improvement in this sleep problem.

Overall, 62% of the subjects reported improvement in sleep over the 12-week study, demonstrating the effectiveness of acupuncture in relieving sleep problems that affect menopausal-transition women.

HEART PALPITATIONS

Heart discomfort and heart palpitations were noted by many of the women, but less than 25% noted significant discomfort. According to Chinese medicine, any disruption in the body can affect the heart and cause these manifestations. During the study, heart problems were observed to occur more frequently during the evening time or at rest. Heart discomfort and heart palpitations were significantly relieved by 68%. They were not identified as a problem by any of the women by the end of the study.

JOINT AND MUSCULAR DISCOMFORT

Most women in the study noted minor aches and pains, arthralgia, fibromyalgia, or headaches to some degree on the MRS. It is difficult to know for sure if these symptoms are truly associated with menopausal transition or are more general in nature. Women were excluded from participation if their primary complaints were joint and muscular discomfort and they were not experiencing any of the other common menopausal-transition symptoms.

Women in the study noticed a decrease in joint and muscular discomfort. It is worth noting that joint and muscular discomfort disrupts sleep patterns and increases stress and emotional patterns, thus increasing score levels. Treating women with a chief complaint of joint and muscular discomfort can indirectly affect other common menopausal-transition symptoms.

Psychological Symptoms: Results and Clinical Observations

EMOTIONAL ISSUES

Depression, irritability, and anxiety were closely observed and were identified as significant problems for women in the research study. The reported frequency of emotional issues was similar to the frequency of hot flashes; Chinese medicine describes the connections between the two issues.

The symptoms that responded best in the emotional issues category were depressive symptoms, with treatment effectiveness at 64%

reduction, due to the calming and soothing functions of acupuncture. Irritability reduced by 62%, while the reduction in severity of anxiety was 60%. Anxiety responded slowly and gradually, similar to the improvement in hot flashes.

MENTAL AND PHYSICAL EXHAUSTION

Almost every woman in the study indicated problems with fatigue—mental or physical exhaustion. Even though they are not necessarily considered a chief complaint of menopausal transition, these manifestations received very high ratings on the MRS.

The end results were remarkable, with an overall 64% reduction. By the end of the study, most women did not consider these symptoms to be problems and enjoyed increased energy and clearer thinking.

It is worth noting that the speed at which the women experienced relief in emotional issues was greatly affected by patient diet and exercise habits. Women with poor dietary habits or infrequent activity improved more slowly than women with a balanced diet and exercise routine.

Urogenital Symptoms: Results and Clinical Observations

UROGENITAL DISORDERS

Urogenital disorders encompass: sexual problems, such as libido and satisfaction; bladder problems, such as difficulty urinating, increased need to urinate, and incontinence; vaginal disorders, including dryness, burning, and difficulty with intercourse.

It is worth noting that some women had difficulty with and were apprehensive about discussing these types of issues, especially with a male doctor. With this in mind, MRS scores may have been slightly higher with a female doctor present to discuss these specific issues.

The root cause for most urogenital disorders is kidney essence deficiency or blood deficiency, in conjunction with either kidney yin deficiency or kidney yang deficiency. Sexual problems primarily indicated in the study were low libido and low satisfaction, with subjects presenting with kidney yin deficiency and signs of empty heat. In Chinese medicine, low libido and sexual satisfaction are kidney yang deficiency issues, with desire not being stirred due to a low mingmen fire. This confirms the theory that deficiency of kidney yin or kidney yang, over time, will invariably create deficiency of the other. Women with sexual problems and vaginal dryness issues scored similarly, with a 63% reduction following the acupuncture treatment.

The most noted bladder issue was increase in urgency and frequency and was seen in subjects with both yin and yang deficiency. The pathogenesis is kidney yang unable to warm and support the bladder, thus losing its ability to hold urine and stimulating frequent and urgent urination. Also, excess and deficiency heat symptoms can agitate the lower jiao and bladder, causing an increased need to urinate. With the combination of the two, it is natural for menopausal-transition women to begin having these types of problems. Through the treatment course, there was a 79% decrease in bladder disorders, showing significant success with acupuncture.

Menstrual Irregularities: Results and Clinical Observations

Even though menstrual irregularities are not listed and scored on the MRS, they are frequently a major concern of women in menopausal transition.

Many women in the research suffered from menstrual problems, including irregular menstrual cycles, heavy periods, or not having a period every month. They were assured that this is completely normal during menopausal transition. Most women had no complaints in this area by the end of the treatment sessions.

Heavy, prolonged, or continuous bleeding is a medical concern if the bleeding does not stop. This was observed with four women in the study, with a combined pattern of primary qi deficiency, kidney essence deficiency, and internal heat due to stagnation. After the 12-week treatment course, the menstrual bleeding was controlled in all four women.

Conclusion

Acupuncture treatment has good therapeutic effectiveness in treating menopausal-transition symptoms. It carries low risk, and is minimally invasive, cost effective, and an excellent alternative to standard methods of treatment.

Quantity and Frequency of Treatments

It is difficult to answer when a patient asks how many treatments it will take before their hot flashes go away. Even when the case seems easy, it is best to be cautious when answering. Sometimes hot flashes are quickly and easily abated, while at other times nothing can quell them. The answer is that no two women will respond in the same way. There are many reasons why a case will respond in one way or another.

Typically, the number of treatments required for good resolution depends on whether the patient's hot flashes are in the mild, moderate, or severe category. Ranking hot-flash severity takes into account the patient's health history, constitution, and lifestyle habits, whether they seem deficient or excessive, and the clinician's diagnostic skills.

Average menopausal-transition hot-flash patients tend to rate either in the mild or moderate category, with some cases teetering on the line between moderate and severe. As a clinician, I've found that patients in this category would rather hear they are in the moderate to severe category than in the severe category. Hope can play an important role in creating an optimistic mindset to allow healing. A bit of relaxation can make the treatment process easier and shorter.

Patients falling into the severe category usually have preexisting or extenuating circumstances that amplify their hot flashes. Patients in this category may have any or all of the following: a history of chronic or intractable hot flashes; accompanying fibromyalgia or arthritic pain; pharmaceutical-induced hot flashes; surgical-induced hot flashes; history of severe physical or mental illness; extended drug or pharmaceutical abuse.

Severe hot-flash cases are difficult to treat and tend to show slower rates of improvement. Identifying severe cases allows the practitioner to put in place necessary patient support and make treatment preparations. There is no fast track to relief in many severe cases. Acupuncture will have no effect on a small percentage of severe hot-flash patients.

Quality-of-Life Indicator

Hot flashes normally do not go away entirely after a series of acupuncture treatments, but patients experience significant improvements in their quality of life as the hot flashes subside in severity, frequency, and duration. For most patients, the final result depends on age and where they fall along the menopausal-transition timeline. The goal is to quell and control the hot flashes, not to eliminate them altogether.

Practitioners can utilize a 1–10 scale (1 = mild, 10 = extreme) to track the severity of the patient's hot flashes. When the patient reaches a point where they are comfortable that their hot flashes are manageable, it is called the quality-of-life threshold. For most women, this will be achieved when the rating is reduced to 2–3.

Recovery Rates

The speed of recovery and the extent of relief can vary significantly depending on the woman's diet, ability to deal with stress, rest, and exercise habits. These guidelines provide reasonable estimates for answering patients' questions regarding how many treatments and how long it will take to treat their hot flashes. The quantity and frequency of treatments are based on the severity and duration of the hot-flash symptoms.

- Mild conditions: 3–6 treatments.

- Moderate conditions: 6–12 treatments.

- Severe conditions: 12–24+ treatments.

- Short duration/acute conditions: 3–12 treatments.

- Long duration/chronic conditions: 12–24+ treatments.

- Mild conditions: 1 treatment per week.

- Moderate conditions: 1–2 treatments per week.

- Severe conditions: 2 treatments per week.

- Short duration/acute conditions: 2 treatments per week.

- Long duration/chronic conditions: 1 treatment per week.

When they have reached the quality-of-life threshold, patients will need to continue routine treatments to maintain their quality of life. Maintenance treatments one to two times per month will typically be sufficient to sustain the gains made previously, though some may require more or fewer depending on their particular circumstances.

Patients who have the time and financial means to come in more frequently, especially at the beginning, generally do respond and reach their quality-of-life threshold at a faster pace.

Success Rates

Successful hot-flash treatment with acupuncture depends on many factors. Success sometimes depends on whether or not the patient is able to complete their treatments. Some patients will stop treatments based on time and financial limitations, while others are simply impatient, dislike the treatments, or don't believe that they will work. Some patients simply do not have the patience to accept a realistic timeline for treatment and do not like hearing that it may take several weeks to curb their hot flashes and that to maintain the improvements may require indefinite maintenance treatments.

Success sometimes comes down to the skill level of the practitioner and the support system the practitioner creates for the patient. Based on a great deal of clinical evidence and research, I created the 50%–70%–90%–100% outcome theory. This describes the clinical efficacy of acupuncture in treating hot flashes.

I have found that about 50% of all hot-flash patients will naturally respond to acupuncture treatments with full efficacy results. About 20% will respond more slowly and at a more gradual rate. They will benefit from herbal formulas and modifying lifestyle changes. An additional 20% will need longer treatment courses and it will be necessary for them to take herbal formulas and make lifestyle changes to achieve satisfactory results. The final 10% will not respond to Chinese medicine.

It is relatively easy for a practitioner of any skill level to obtain a

50% success rate with a standard course of acupuncture. Just insert needles, repeat, and watch the patient get results. A 50% success rate, however, is also a 50% failure rate! No practitioner should be willing to accept that level of performance.

It's not very difficult to increase clinical outcomes to 70% and help more patients. This requires study to gain additional knowledge and the application of lessons learned from clinical experience. It requires improved acupuncture techniques and knowing how to adjust point prescriptions. It requires being able to identify which herbal formulas will best address a woman's hot-flash environment. Most seasoned acupuncturists meet these criteria.

Raising clinical efficacy to 90% is a true challenge. In the realm of treating menopausal transition and hot flashes, to truly be able to help the most difficult patients takes time, understanding, and effort. The clinician at this point must learn from the patient. It is vital to question why the patient is not responding and explore alternatives. The practitioner must pay attention to messages the patient's body is sending. This is where the real clinical magic happens. As healers, we are only as good as the most difficult cases we are able to treat.

Treatment Schedule

Setting up a treatment schedule is a good idea for two reasons. First, it will help track how well the patient is responding and measure the clinical efficacy of the acupuncture treatments. Second, it will serve as a learning guide for the practitioner.

Consistency is important. If treatment modalities are frequently changed—different acupuncture prescriptions, herbal prescriptions, and lifestyle changes—then the practitioner has no way of knowing what has actually been effective.

The first step in establishing a treatment plan is to prescribe a set number of treatments and a treatment schedule based on the severity of the patient's hot-flash environment. Be confident and assured. Gain the trust of the patient.

Next, set up an acupuncture protocol and point prescription based on the initial diagnosis. Is it an excess or deficient hot-flash environment? Try keeping everything simple. Stick to a general acupuncture prescription.

Avoid prescribing herbal formulas when initiating treatment unless you are certain of a particular need. Be mindful about suggesting too many lifestyle changes. The objective is to have control of the treatment environment. Too many variables will lead to confusion. Herbal formulas and lifestyle suggestions can be added as treatment progresses, when the practitioner feels they are appropriate.

As treatment proceeds, note changes in hot-flash severity, duration, frequency, and other menopausal symptoms. If the patient is responding, continue along with the treatment schedule. Once the patient's symptoms are manageable and their quality-of-life parameters have been met, adjust the frequency of the treatments appropriately.

If there are no changes after a certain amount of treatments, modify the acupuncture prescription and repeat. Ideally, the patient should start seeing and feeling results after three treatments in mild cases, six to nine treatments in moderate cases, and nine to twelve treatments in severe cases. If there are no changes after the set treatment course, reassess and start a new treatment schedule along with changes in herbal-formula prescriptions and lifestyle modifications.

Clinical Hot-Flash Point Prescriptions
The Constitutions: Treating a Deficiency or Excess Hot-Flash Environment

It is normal to start treating most hot-flash patients with either an excess or deficiency acupuncture prescription based on the initial patient intake and diagnosis. Excess or deficiency acupuncture prescriptions can and should be modified based on the patient's need and current presentations.

There are many acupuncture prescriptions and possible combinations that will be effective. I have developed these acupuncture prescriptions over many years of treating many patients, learning from both successes and failures. I find the excess or deficiency acupuncture prescriptions quite effective.

I modify the acupuncture formulas over time after monitoring the changes and outcomes in the individual patient. This is based on what improves, what doesn't change, and what gets worse. Over time, points are modified, tried, and proven, or sometimes adjusted according to what gets worse. Patients will begin to settle into their unique points that you find are clinically proven to work for them. The excess and deficiency prescriptions are a starting point.

Deficiency-Patterns Point Prescription

When treating hot flashes with acupuncture, it is necessary to support pre-heaven and post-heaven qi. This provides continual nourishment for the zangfu organs, especially the heart, and allows essence to be built up and stored in the kidney. It is also essential to sedate hyperactive yang qi, quell fire, and soothe qi stagnation, which protects the heart from harassment.

This well-rounded acupuncture prescription is a slight adjustment to the prescription used for my original research, eliminating PC6 and adding DU24. The aim is to balance yin and yang, and reestablish a working zangfu organ and channel system to treat the hot-flash environment: DU20 (Baihui) 百会, DU24 (Shenting) 神庭, HT7 (Shenmen) 神门, LI4 (Hegu) 合谷, RN6 (Qihai) 气海, RN4 (Guanyuan) 关元, ST36 (Zusanli) 足三里, SP6 (Sanyinjiao) 三阴交, KI3 (Taixi) 太溪, and LR3 (Taichong) 太冲.

This is a gathering of some of the most commonly used and powerful acupuncture points on the body. Its main focus is to balance yin and yang between the upper and lower triads by tonifying and nourishing essence, yin, and blood in the lower kidney-liver-spleen triad, and regulating yang qi, stagnation, and heat in the upper liver-spleen-heart triad. It is ideally suited to the deficiency environments with concurrent excess symptoms often seen in the clinical setting.

NEEDLE INSERTION

I generally begin needling the dantian on the abdomen at RN6 and RN4. This is the center of the body and the origin of the essential (jing) qi. Needling here first stimulates the mingmen, which is host to the kidney essence, yin, and true yang situated between the kidneys. This sets the intention for the rest of the treatment.

This serves as the foundation for source (yuan) qi. Once needled, subsequent acupuncture points can then establish communication from the mingmen to the zangfu organs and tissues. RN6 and RN4 serve as the fuse box, the channel system serves as the wiring, subsequent points serve as the on/off switches, and the zangfu organs serve as the lights and appliances.

Next, I move on to the legs and needle ST36, SP6, KI3, and LR3. These points support the kidney, liver, and spleen's ability to preserve essence, fortify yuan qi, and generate new qi and blood. I needle bilaterally and generally from the knee distally towards the ankles. LR3 is needled last to allow more time for the channels to fill before the qi soothing function of LR3 is administered. I may switch to alternative points along these channels, depending on the patient's overall sensitivity to stimulation.

Treating points on the upper (yang) extremities following the treatment of points on the lower (yin) extremities allows yin to build before yang is set in motion. I first needle HT7 to bring the awareness to the heart, which in turn establishes the connection between the mingmen and the heart. LI4 is administered after HT7. LI4 has the ability to launch the powerful yin and yang qi connections throughout the body. It is like flipping on the main switch to the system and brings awareness and balance to the nervous system.

I finish the treatments at the head. DU24 is needled first and acts as an equalizer by smoothing qi and blood flow throughout the body. The last point is DU20 at the crown of the head. This point establishes yin and yang balance within the blood, channels, and zangfu organ system.

RN6 (Qihai) 气海

RN6 is known as the "sea of qi," and primarily functions to tonify source (yuan) qi and the kidney. The yuan qi, which comes from the pre-heaven and post-heaven qi, is the source of nourishment for the entire body. RN6 is also known for its ability to move qi and is often selected for qi stagnation in the lower abdomen.

It is necessary to continually support yuan qi during the aging process for overall longevity purposes. It is easy to understand why utilizing RN6 is warranted in treating general deficiency issues and during the menopausal transition process. RN6 is especially useful in nourishing and supplying qi and blood to the heart and brain for mental and physical fatigue.

RN4 (Guanyuan) 关元

RN4 is known as the "source gate" and is an indispensable point to fortify source (yuan) qi, nourish kidney essence, support the uterus, and regulate the lower jiao. Source gate refers to this point being the essential acupuncture point on the body used to stimulate the source (yuan) qi stored and generated within the dantian. This vital qi serves as the foundation or "source" of life.

RN4 strengthens and improves hormonal imbalances and treats hot flashes, palpitations, and night sweats by harmonizing the heart fire and kidney water. It is also used for treating common menstrual and urogenital disorders during menopausal transition.

RN4 and RN6 are a common dual point combination located on the dantian. RN6 assists the yang within yin function by generating qi and fortifying yang, while RN4 assists the yin within yin function by nourishing blood and yin.

Yuan qi is the fuel for the body. Stimulating various acupoints without supporting the yuan qi is like maintaining a fire by blowing on it but not adding more wood. It is absolutely necessary to needle RN4 and RN6 when treating the hot-flash environment. In certain excess hot-flash environments, RN6 is too yang qi stimulating and should be omitted.

Both acupoints are easy to needle and carry little risk but are susceptible to needle sensitivity in thin patients. If this is the case, a gentle, inferior oblique or transverse insertion is warranted.

ST36 (Zusanli) 足三里

ST36 is arguably the most commonly used acupoint on the body. Its primary function is to tonify qi and blood by strengthening the spleen and stomach. This means that ST36 is a primary acupoint for the generation of the zhen qi. With this, it can regulate the nourishing functions of ying qi and protective and warming functions of wei qi.

Hot flashes and various menopausal-transition symptoms can result if ying qi falls deficient or if wei qi becomes erratic.

With its tonifying ability, ST36 is able to treat a wide variety of manifestations attributed to menopausal transition including fatigue, heart palpitations, insomnia, sweating issues, emotional imbalances, and menstrual irregularities.

ST36 is not only able to nourish qi and blood, it is also able to clear fire from the yangming channels. Excess fire can travel via the stomach channel to harass the heart fire and overstimulate the brain, which makes ST36 capable of relieving hot flashes, insomnia, and depression seen in menopausal-transition women.

My professor Dr. Fei Xiao called Zusanli "the everything point" and said one could use it for treating any condition. I administer ST36 for most hot-flash situations presenting with an underlying deficiency pattern, even when excessive symptoms are present.

There are two conditions for which I do not use ST36: pure excessive patterns or acupuncture hypersensitivity. In excessive situations, it is suitable to select alternative acupoints or simply utilize a different point on the channel such as ST44 (Neiting) (内庭).

It is difficult to needle at ST36 on some menopausal-transition patients with increased acupuncture sensitivity. There are two primary reasons for this. First, the peroneal (deep branch) nerve runs below ST36 and is easily stimulable in hypersensitive patients.

Second, women may hold body fluids and have swelling, especially in the lower leg region, whether due to hormone fluctuations or as a result of diet and lifestyle issues. Fluid accumulation creates pressure and tightness in the calf region and on the peroneal and local cutaneous nerves. Strong qi sensation in this situation increases fluid pressure on the nerve, creating pain and nerve discomfort. If it is absolutely essential to use ST36, switching to a 38-gauge needle and using gentle insertion at a shallower depth with less qi sensation is warranted.

SP6 (Sanyinjiao) 三阴交
SP6 is the crossing point of the spleen, liver, and kidney yin channels, hence its name "three yin crossing." One can simultaneously treat these three zangfu organs by needling this one point. It benefits the

spleen, tonifies the kidney, nourishes liver blood, and supports the kidney-liver-spleen triad.

SP6 has a strong commanding action to carry out its duties. Not only does it produce and preserve pre-heaven and post-heaven qi, but it also produces qi, blood, and essence to spread and nourish the entire zangfu organ system and tissues throughout the body.

SP6 is an indispensable point for treating hot flashes and menopausal-transition symptoms with its wide, versatile range of actions. It can be used in almost every situation.

Much like ST36, there are some circumstances when it is not appropriate to utilize SP6. Acupuncture hypersensitivity or nerve hyper-stimulability are contraindications to utilizing SP6. The tibia nerve runs anterior to this point and can be activated to stimulate strong muscle aches or nerve pain in the local area. This can happen with an incorrect insertion angle or deep needling, or in some patients where the nerve innervation is shallow or more posterior than normal. Problems with utilizing SP6 are more common in thinner patients.

SP6 has a strong commanding action in generating and moving qi and blood. This is not warranted and further agitates some hot-flash environments with presentations of excess yang qi, fire, or stagnation. SP9 is a good alternative on the spleen channel in these circumstances. SP3 is a good alternative in cases of pure qi deficiency.

KI3 (Taixi) 太溪

KI3 is the yuan-source point on the kidney channel and is designated to tonify and nourish the kidney in its entirety including yin, yang, and essence, deeming it the most adaptable acupoint on the kidney channel.

KI3 is an indispensable point for treating hot flashes and menopausal-transition symptoms, with its wide, versatile range of actions. It can be used in almost every situation. KI3 is especially useful for regulating and reestablishing the kidney's relationship with the other zang organs.

The kidney has an intimate connection with every zangfu organ. There is a kidney deficiency component in every hot-flash environment. It is necessary to support the kidney to maintain balance throughout the system.

The kidney and heart control the sovereign and ministerial fire and together they mutually warm the zangfu organs and power the activity in the body. However, it is easy for the two to fall out of balance during menopausal transition, thus creating disequilibrium between water and fire or yin and yang.

Kidney essence is the foundation of liver blood. The kidney and liver become increasingly depleted of essence and blood throughout the aging process. It is necessary to continuously nourish the two during menopausal transition. When both organs are healthy, together the kidney and liver can balance yin and yang qi.

The kidney and spleen work together to maintain and preserve the pre-heaven and post-heaven qi. The kidney preserves itself by supporting the spleen's function of transformation and transportation, and, together, the kidney and spleen supply qi and blood to the entire body.

The kidney and lung maintain proper breath, qi, and blood circulation, and together they maintain harmony and protect the zangfu organ system from decline and dysfunction.

It is easy to incorporate multiple needles along the kidney channel during a treatment to enhance the desired function. For example, administering KI2 along with KI3 has a stronger action in terms of quelling heart fire. The two work together and enhance the ability to control water and fire balance to relieve hot flashes.

One caution: strong stimulation and incorrect needling technique can disturb the tibia nerve, which lies directly below KI3, creating a strong electrical response that will radiate down into the arch and sole of the foot.

LR3 (Taichong) 太冲

LR3 is the yuan-source point on the liver channel and has the actions of nourishing liver yin and blood, regulating yin and yang, and soothing liver qi. It is necessary to support all of these functions to maintain a healthy menopausal transition.

LR3 has the unique ability to regulate every aspect of the excess and deficiency hot-flash environment created by the consumption of yin, blood, and essence, and the generation of hyperactive yang qi, fire, and stagnation. These imbalances are the root cause of hot flashes and most menopausal-transition symptoms, including anxiety, depression, fatigue, insomnia, and gynecological and urogenital disorders.

The liver is classically known as holding a position in the lower jiao along with the kidney and alternatively holding a position in the middle jiao along with the spleen. The liver forms unique relationships with the kidney and spleen.

As described previously, the liver and kidney share the duty of balancing yin and yang. They are both susceptible to yin deficiency, leading to deficiency fire and hyperactive yang rising. LR3, with its dual ability to nourish and drain, treats yin deficiency, subdues yang qi, and quells fire. This is a typical hot-flash scenario.

The liver (wood) and spleen (earth) share a five-phase relationship that is susceptible to imbalance. It is easy for the liver to become excessive and overactive from daily stress and emotional instability. On the other side, it is easy for the spleen to become weak and submissive from rumination and irregular dietary habits. Either of the two situations creates an imbalance of the two organs, resulting in the spleen's inability to adequately produce qi and blood and the liver's inability to soothe the movement of qi. This too is a typical hot-flash scenario. My professor Dr. Qiu Hua Shan taught me to always use LR3 to regulate the liver and spleen for this precise reason.

There is a misconception among acupuncturists that LR3 moves qi and blood greatly and therefore should only be needled when there is stagnation or stasis. I believe this notion is primarily based on the "four-gates" theory, the acupuncture point combination where LR3 is needled along with LI4 to treat pain due to channel obstruction. The true action of LR3 resides in the intention of the clinician, supporting acupuncture points, and needling techniques. As the yuan-source point, LR3 is the primary acupuncture point to support the liver.

Point location and needling strength can cause discomfort for the patient. Be sure that the needle insertion is clearly in the soft tissue center between the first and second metatarsals. Strong stimulation or improper location can generate pain or stimulate the deep peroneal nerve branches located bilaterally beneath this point. It may be necessary to use a 38-gauge needle for acupuncture with hypersensitive patients.

HT7 (Shenmen) 神门

The heart is the monarch of the zangfu organs and the governor of blood. HT7 is the yuan-source point on the heart channel and has the actions of nourishing the heart and calming the spirit, whether there is excess or deficiency.

The heart spirit desires tranquility, and to accomplish this it requires an abundant supply of qi, blood, yin, and yang from the spleen, liver, and kidney. The heart becomes deficient when the supply chain is disrupted due to deficiency or blocked because of stagnation.

When the heart becomes deficient, it manifests and amplifies menopausal-transition symptoms such as hot flashes, insomnia, palpitations, and anxiety. The nourishing action of HT7 supports the heart's reception of qi and blood from the other organs to treat these issues.

Heart fire is kept in check by a healthy balance of yin (water) from the kidney. This is the principal mechanism of the hot-flash environment. The heart fire is susceptible to harassment from hyperactive yang rising or exuberant fire. Either situation will cause the heart fire to flare up, giving rise to the classic hot-flash scenario. HT7 has a unique ability to abate blazing heart fire and quell hot flashes.

The ulnar nerve lies beneath HT7. Directing the needle angle slightly laterally will lessen the chances of nerve stimulation. For patients retaining body fluids due to hormonal changes, yin excess, or yin fire, HT7 may be more problematic to needle because fluid pressure will allow the needle sensation to overstimulate the nerve. Utilizing a 38-gauge needle or selecting HT6 or HT3 will avoid this issue.

LI4 (Hegu) 合谷

LI4 is a well-known pain-relief acupressure point and is widely used for both its analgesic and sedative effects. For this reason, LI4 is arguably one of the most commonly researched acupuncture points. It has a wide-reaching range of actions for treating pain and neurological disorders with its influencing nature on the nervous system.

Based on its neurological efficacy, it is especially useful for treating hot flashes and other menopausal-transition symptoms. LI4 has both stimulating and sedating effects on the brain and directly accesses the HPO axis to regulate thermoregulation. This is supported by LI4 being known as one of the best acupuncture points for treating head disorders.

In Chinese medicine, LI4 functions to calm the mind to induce relaxation. This is especially useful for many patients with anxiety and stress patterns.

LI4 is one of the best points for regulating wei qi and sweating issues. This point controls body temperature with its ability to regulate the opening and closing of sweat pores. LI4 is often combined with points like ST36, LU7, KI7, KI6, and HT6 for treating various types of sweating disorder based on pattern differentiation.

LI4 promotes smooth circulation of qi and blood when used in conjunction with LR3. Known as the "four gates" together, they regulate circulating qi and blood through the channels to relieve qi stagnation related issues and are able to treat menopausal-transition fatigue and pain-related issues.

LI4 is a highly sensitive acupuncture point. When needled incorrectly, it will elicit discomfort and pain. This is common when locating it at the highest point of the dorsal interosseous muscle. It is less sensitive when it is needled slightly closer to the second metatarsal bone. Acupuncture-sensitive patients will respond better to a slower and gentler insertion technique and the use of 38-gauge needles. If it is too sensitive, using this point can be counterproductive as it can overstimulate the nervous system.

DU20 (Baihui) 百会

DU20 is a transporting point for the sea of marrow and functions to nourish and benefit the brain, regulate ascending yang, and calm the shen. This acupoint is the direct spark for the brain.

The brain (yang) is the sea of marrow and is directly connected to the kidney (yin) essence. The governing vessel (du mai) connects the two. The governing vessel governs yang qi and is counterbalanced by the conception vessel (ren mai), which governs yin qi.

Yang qi helps transform kidney (yin) essence within the mingmen and then ascend newly formed essence to fill the sea of marrow. Without the governing vessel, kidney essence would stay in the depths of the mingmen.

The sea of marrow relies on essence for proper mental function, which translates as proper brain and neuro-endocrine function. This is why it is essential to continuously nourish the kidney and fortify yang qi.

This rise and fall of yin and yang is the prerequisite for life. DU20 establishes and regulates this function. The HPO axis depends on the balance of yin and yang. During the aging process and especially menopausal transition, it's natural for the yin to become increasingly deficient, leaving the sea of marrow malnourished. Along with this process, unabated yang qi becomes hyperactive. This creates the perfect hot-flash environment, an undernourished and overstimulated neuro-endocrine system.

DU20 regulates yang qi, which means it stimulates weakness and sedates excess. It is utilized to stimulate and raise essence to the sea of marrow and to calm hyperactivity within the brain. It is a simplistic misconception that DU20 only stimulates yang qi to rise. If yang qi is too hyperactive, DU20 will sedate and redirect it downward.

By supporting the connection between the sea of marrow and kidney and balancing of yin and yang qi, DU20 is able to calm the spirit and treat menopausal-transition symptoms such as hot flashes, headache, dizziness, poor memory, insomnia, and anxiety.

DU24 (Shenting) 神庭

DU24 is named the "spirit courtyard" and highlights its function to calm the shen. This point is used purely to calm the nervous system to enhance relaxation and vital qi regeneration.

DU24 is especially useful for treating hot flashes, with its ability to calm the mind. Calming the spirit functions to sedate hyperactive yang qi and soothe qi flow, which opens up thermoregulation. This simple function conducted over and over regulates and supports the HPO axis through menopausal transition. When set into motion, the correct internal zangfu organ environment is reestablished, which allows for generation of fresh qi and blood and essence reserves to be built back up.

DU20 and DU24 are relatively easy to needle. A posterior insertion is common when the patient is in a supine position. Needle depth depends on the patient; it can be inserted up to 1.5 cun or inches if desired. Sensitivity increases with dehydrated patients, and discomfort increases if insertion is too shallow.

The shen calming effectiveness of DU20 and DU24 can be enhanced with the use of acupuncture electrostimulation. A low-frequency (2–5 hertz) continuous dense wave is preferred, with the positive electrode connected to DU20 and the negative electrode connected to DU24. Electro-acupuncture from DU20 to DU24 is particularly effective in treating intractable insomnia cases.

Excess-Patterns Point Prescription

Treating hot flashes in a relative excess hot-flash environment takes a different approach to that used for treating deficiency patterns. It is one of draining, sedating, and clearing while providing continual support to the pre-heaven and post-heaven qi. Without this simultaneous effort, qi and blood will remain stagnant, damaged, and deficient, and the hot flashes will eventually return.

The following excess hot-flash acupuncture prescription modifies the formula from my original research by changing two points along the spleen and stomach channel, eliminating RN6, and adding regulating points on the pericardium and gallbladder channels: DU20 (Baihui) 百会, DU24 (Shenting) 神庭, HT7 (Shenmen) 神门, PC6 (Neiguan) 内关, LI4 (Hegu) 合谷, RN4 (Guanyuan) 关元, ST44 (Neiting) 内庭, SP9 (Yinlingquan) 阴陵泉, KI3 (Taixi) 太溪, LR3 (Taichong) 太冲, and GB34 (Yanglingquan) 阳陵泉.

This point prescription is especially useful for the hot-flash patient presenting with relative excess symptoms on top of a weakened constitution. It is also particularly effective for the needle-sensitive or hypersensitive acupuncture patient.

NEEDLE INSERTION

The order for needle insertion for excess patterns is similar to that described for deficiency patterns. As previously described, RN6 can stoke and stir yang qi and is omitted for excess hot-flash environments. The primary focus on the lower abdomen is on RN4 to support deficiency to allow yin and yang to regain balance once the excess is cleared. RN3 should be used instead of RN4 in cases of yin fire or damp-heat accumulation in the lower jiao.

The insertion order on the leg channels is similar, starting at the knee and working inferiorly down towards the foot. This serves two purposes. First, SP9 and GB34 are generally less needle sensitive. Second, they stabilize qi and blood within the leg channels to allow for the stronger actions of LR3 or ST44. The final points on the upper extremities and head are treated the same as in the previous prescription.

SP9 (Yinlingquan) 阴陵泉

The spleen channel can become excessive in some excess hot-flash environments, even when the spleen organ itself is weak. Whether this is due to internal yin fire or stagnation issues, it is necessary to drain the spleen channel. SP6 is a miraculous acupoint with the ability to resolve many spleen issues; however, its qi and blood nourishing and moving functions will agitate an excess state.

SP9 is the he-sea point on the spleen channel and primarily functions to drain excess dampness generated by spleen deficiency. When dampness accumulates, it has the tendency to create qi stagnation and heat. This is why SP9 is an effective point. It not only drains the dampness, but it also drains heat and unblocks the qi.

Finally, he-sea points support their corresponding zangfu organs even though they are not commonly thought of as tonification points. This gives the practitioner the opportunity to simultaneously drain excess and nourish deficiency. He-sea points are located around the knees and elbows and are less susceptible to needle sensitivity than their yuan-source point counterparts located around the wrists.

GB34 (Yanglingquan) 阳陵泉

The gallbladder and san jiao shaoyang are qi regulation channels. Regulation describes their ability to rectify disproportionate qi and blood, yin and yang, excess and deficiency, and interior and exterior issues throughout the body. The strong actions of GB34 can carry out these regulation activities because the gallbladder channel navigates the internal and external body from head to toe.

GB34 primarily functions to regulate qi and blood and clear heat due to stagnation issues. GB34 can be thought of as a complementary or supporting point where it serves to enhance the actions of the rest of the prescription.

ST44 (Neiting) 内庭

ST44 is the first ying-spring point formally being introduced for treating the hot-flash environment. The primary function of all ying-spring points is simply to clear heat and fire and they are suitable for excess and deficiency patterns. The stomach yangming channel is prone to excess qi and blood and heat repletion. The stomach divergent channel directly links to the heart. Any heat repletion in the stomach channel can directly harass the heart fire.

ST44 serves two important functions in treating hot flashes. It opens and allows excess heat to drain from the channel, allowing excess heart fire to drain as well. It also has a strong shen calming action. This dual action reduces harassment and provides a calm environment for the heart.

Needle insertion at ST44 can be somewhat alarming for some patients. It is good practice to tell the patient before insertion that this point may elicit a quick sting or nerve twinge. To lessen discomfort, be sure to needle into the soft flesh just distally between the two joints and not into the periosteum of either joint causing sharp pain.

PC6 (Neiguan) 内关

PC6 is a versatile point for treating hot flashes and menopausal transition. The pericardium and liver jueyin channels regulate qi and blood and balance yin and yang qi. Together, they function to control hyperactive or ascending yang qi and fire due to deficiency, excess, or stagnation situations.

Jueyin channels function more on the yang aspects of qi, while their shaoyin channel counterparts (heart and kidney) focus more on the yin aspects of qi. This is why PC6 and HT7 are an effective yin and yang point combination. They have a dual nourishing and clearing action for treating hot flashes and other heart symptoms, such as insomnia, anxiety, depression, and palpitations, frequently seen in menopausal-transition patients.

PC6 has a strong regulating function in the chest and upper abdomen and is able to clear excess heart fire and calm the heart spirit. PC6 is more suited to treating excess conditions, while its counterpart, HT7, is more suited to nourishing deficiency.

PC6 is widely known for its ability to direct counterflow qi downwards. Counterflow or rebellious qi is often seen in pregnancy, menopausal transition, and anxiety patients. It happens when ascendant liver qi is too strong due to yin deficiency, hyperactive yang, or blazing yin fire, causing excessive qi to rise up through the kidney, stomach, and chong channels. It can also happen when lung and stomach qi are stagnant and unable to descend, and they stagnate in the chest and diaphragm. Ascending yang, fire, or stagnation from any of these scenarios will harass and agitate the heart. PC6 is remarkable for treating all types of counterflow qi disorders.

PC6 is the confluent point of the yinwei mai. It is paired with SP4, the confluent point of the chong mai. This special relationship allows PC6 the ability to redirect ascending surging qi or fire due to various menopausal-transition patterns downwards, thus treating hot flashes, anxiety, and insomnia.

PC6 is a challenging point to administer because the median nerve lies beneath it and is easily stimulable. Utilizing a transverse insertion will lessen the chances of causing strong nerve stimulation.

Like HT7, patients retaining body fluids can make PC6 problematic to needle because of fluid pressure on the nerve. Utilizing gentle needling techniques or using 38-gauge needles may lessen the chances of nerve stimulation.

Hot-Flash Acupuncture Modifications

It is not necessary to adhere strictly to either the deficiency or excess hot-flash acupuncture prescriptions. Acupuncture and Chinese medicine are living and breathing medicines tailored to meet the needs and requirements of the individual patient. In many cases, it will be necessary to modify one of the prescriptions.

Hot-flash acupuncture modifications have been divided into three sections—acupuncture points for: clearing heat and fire; calming the spirit; resolving stagnation issues.

Heat and Fire

It is easy to focus on clearing heat and purging fire when treating hot flashes. It is tempting to adopt an acupuncture prescription around a group of heat clearing points. It is true that sometimes hot flashes do respond well to heat clearing and fire draining points. Most of the time, however, the effects are short lived and the heat returns.

Hot flashes may not be sufficiently relieved through heat clearing acupoints. Hot flashes arise as the manifestation of internal imbalance. It is necessary to address and rectify the underlying pathophysiological aspects creating the heat or fire manifestation. These underlying aspects are addressed with the deficiency and excess acupuncture prescriptions. When warranted, it is necessary to add additional points to the acupuncture prescription that specifically address internal heat and fire.

KI2 (RANGU) 然谷 AND KI6 (ZHAOHAI) 照海

The kidney channel is a primary focus for treating the hot-flash environment. As discussed, KI3 is an indispensable point for treating hot flashes, based on its versatility. Sometimes, though, the internal fire may be too strong for this one point to quell it. It is then necessary to obtain help by selecting another point along the kidney channel. Using another point will amplify the effects of KI3. In this case, two is better than one.

KI2 is a ying-spring point and its primary function is to clear deficiency heat. Its strong ability to quell blazing fire deep within the mingmen is remarkable. The increasing water action of KI3 and fire clearing action of KI2 enhance each other beautifully. Together, they are one of the best two-point acupuncture combinations on the body to quell hot flashes.

KI6 is often touted as the go-to acupoint for clearing deficiency heat, especially for patients suffering from hot flashes. The same is true for HT6. KI6 is the confluent point for the yinqiao mai and is often paired with LU7, the confluent point of the ren mai for treating menopausal transition and its accompanying symptoms.

KI6 functions well to nourish relative yin deficiency throughout the body. Its deficiency heat clearing ability, however, is less than KI2, even when paired with KI3. Long-term menopausal transition and post-menopausal treatments that require continual yin nourishing benefit from the KI6 and KI3 combination.

Needling KI2 is somewhat of an advanced acupuncture technique and requires proper location and a gentle needle insertion. KI2 is located at the height of the medial arch in the soft depression below the navicular bone and above the dense fascia. Needling too close to the bone or into the fascia will cause sharp pain or a strong ache. The tight skin on the side of the foot requires a gentle, quick, and smooth insertion to avoid a sharp or stinging sensation. Switching to a thinner-gauge needle may be challenging, as it may bend or get hung up in the superficial skin layer, especially in patients with tough or tight skin.

KI6 is a relatively easy point to needle. It does require the same gentle, quick, and smooth insertion as KI2 to avoid sharp or stinging sensation. The area around KI6 has an abundance of blood vessels, nerve endings, and tendons. It is quite easy to pierce one from time to time, so be mindful.

HT8 (SHAOFU) 少府 AND HT6 (YINXI) 阴郄
The heart and kidney channels are both shaoyin. The heart and kidney together maintain the yin (water) and yang (fire) balance within the body. The heart governs the sovereign fire and the kidney govern the ministerial fire.

The HT8 and HT6 point pair shares many similarities with the KI2 and KI6 pair. HT8 and KI2 are both ying-spring points and function to clear fire. While KI2 has the ability to clear kidney or mingmen fire, HT8 is able to clear heart fire. HT8 is particularly effective in clearing excess heart fire and calming the spirit in patients with relatively strong hot flashes accompanied by heightened anxiety and stubborn insomnia. HT8 and KI2 can be used together to treat intractable hot flashes.

Unlike KI2 working synergistically with KI3, HT8 is effective on its own and doesn't need to be paired with HT7 for supplementation. This is because the heart is supported and nourished by utilizing points below on the spleen and kidney channels.

HT6, like KI6, has long been thought of as the mandatory acupoint for clearing deficiency heat, especially for patients suffering from hot flashes. HT6 is effective at treating relative heart yin deficiency; however, the difference in clinical efficacy between HT6 and HT7 is not noticeable in treating hot flashes. HT6 is more noted for nourishing yin and heart blood and stopping night sweating. Needling HT6 follows the same techniques as HT7.

HT8 is located on the palm of the hand in the soft depression between the fourth and fifth metacarpal bones. Much like KI2, the tight skin on the palm requires a gentle, quick, and smooth insertion to lessen a sharp or stinging sensation. Any strong qi sensations subside once the needle reaches the appropriate depth. It is good practice to warn your patient before insertion that this point may elicit a quick sting. Remind them to breathe.

PC8 (LAOGONG) 劳宫

Acupoints along the heart and pericardium channels often have similar functions and indications. There is a yin and yang difference between the two. As organs, the pericardium on the outside wraps and protects the sovereign heart on the inside. The pericardium is yang while the heart is yin in function and location. The channels function in a similar way. The heart channel is shaoyin and serves as yin within yin, while the pericardium channel is jueyin and serves as yang within yin.

PC8 is similar to HT8, both being ying-spring points and functioning to clear fire from the heart and pericardium and to calm the spirit. The only difference is PC8 has a stronger ability in quelling intractable blazing fire within the upper and middle jiao.

PC8 is appropriate for intractable hot flashes and insomnia. PC8 can be paired with other points for different effects.

- PC8 and HT8: clears excessive heart fire and sedates the shen in relatively excess patterns.

- PC8 and HT7: simultaneously clears excessive heart fire and nourishes the heart in mutual excess and deficiency patterns.

- PC8 and KI2: clears excessive heart fire along with blazing ministerial fire in both excess and deficiency patterns.

- PC8 and KI1: clears heart fire and strongly sedates the shen in chronic conditions.

Needle insertion techniques for PC8 are the same as for HT8.

LR2 (XINGJIAN) 行间 AND GB43 (XIAXI) 侠溪

The liver and gallbladder are interior-exterior related zangfu organs and are regularly treated together. LR2 and GB43 are both ying-spring points and their primary functions are to clear excess fire or damp-heat from their respective channels and organs.

Liver and gallbladder heat, fire, and damp-heat are often due to qi stagnation generated by pent-up emotions, dietary habits, or various long-standing chronic conditions. This excess situation can easily harass the heart spirit and agitate the heart fire.

Hot flashes tend to flare, are particularly intense at times, and are often seen in younger patients during the earlier stages of menopausal transition with relatively strong constitutions. Patients in this category often have stress, agitation, and temper issues, as well as difficulty falling asleep and staying asleep. It is therefore necessary to add LR2 and GB43 to any prescription in these circumstances. Needle insertion for LR2 and GB43 is the same as ST44.

LI11 (QUCHI) 曲池

LI11 has long been regarded as a general all-purpose heat clearing point. It is traditionally used for fever due to wind-heat invasions from colds and flu. Acupuncture sources state that LI11 has a wide set of heat clearing functions, including heat from all areas and levels of the body.

The large intestine yangming channel is rich in qi and blood and susceptible to replete conditions. This would suggest using LI11 to clear heat as a result of excess patterns. It is easily paired with ST44 on the stomach yangming channel, or paired with ST40 in chronic conditions.

LI11 can clear heat that travels through the yangming channels to harass the heart. Though the large intestine channel does not directly connect to the heart, the stomach yangming channel does have a direct connection. LI11 is able to clear excess heat harassing the heart fire and disturbing the spirit, making it appropriate for hot flashes in a relatively excess hot-flash environment.

LI11 is clinically indicated for treating hypertension where yangming excess is the driving force behind ascending yang qi. LI11 is able to clear the excess but not able to tonify deficiency.

Finally, LI11 can treat a wide variety of skin disorders with its ability to cool blood. It is easy to add this point to any hot-flash prescription for a patient presenting with hot flashes and skin issues and it can be paired with PC3.

LI11 is an easy acupuncture point to locate and administer with few difficulties. The elbow is rich in nerves and blood vessels, which can easily be stimulated with an incorrect location or deep insertion. It is best to needle LI11 with the elbow slightly flexed. It is an effective alternative to LI4 for calming the spirit, especially in hypersensitive patients.

SJ5 (WAIGUAN) 外关

SJ5, like LI11, is traditionally known for its efficacy in clearing relatively superficial heat such as fever due to wind-heat invasions. Wind-heat may aggravate but does not generate hot flashes.

Shaoyang channels are interiorly-exteriorly paired with jueyin channels and are prone to both qi and blood stagnation and heat repletion. SJ5 has the additional function of clearing heat along these channels as a result of knotting or stagnation issues.

San jiao and gallbladder shaoyang channel points may be employed to treat chronic and stubborn cases. SJ5 is often useful for treating long-standing cases of heat that have lodged in the body and won't resolve.

SJ5 is an easy point to locate and needle. The extensor tendons can be highly sensitive in some patients. Clinically, I prefer the stronger clearing-heat and stagnation-resolving function of SJ6 over SJ5 for treating hot flashes.

LU10 (YUJI) 鱼际

LU10 is sometimes listed in tidal heat effusion acupuncture prescriptions. I have not used it extensively, nor have I seen any particular efficacy in its use for treating hot flashes. I hypothesize that its ability to quell hot flashes is because it is the ying-spring point on the lung channel, and its ability to clear excess and deficiency heat from the lung and chest make it capable of calming the spirit and quelling hot flashes. The lung is light in nature and positioned in the chest. LU10 can clear heat and fire in the chest but is less effective in treating the root cause of the hot-flash environment. LU10 has little ability in tonify deficiency or resolving stagnation issues.

LU10 has a strong qi sensation and is a sensitive acupoint, so the practitioner must give serious consideration to the challenges versus potential benefits before adding it to the prescription. LU10 is needled in the soft tissue between the first metacarpal bone and the thenar muscle. It requires a gentle needling approach or using 38-gauge needles to lessen patient discomfort.

SP10 (XUEHAI) 血海

SP10 is not commonly used to address hot flashes but can be an effective addition to any hot-flash prescription when there are significant blood stasis and heat patterns.

Qi and blood circulation becomes more erratic in the chong mai, liver, and uterus during the earlier stages of menopausal transition. SP10 is very useful for patients when the menstrual cycle is irregular, heavy, and erratic. It resolves these issues by smoothing the flow of qi and blood and clearing heat.

The spleen is able to generate new blood. Heat is relieved once stagnation is resolved and blood can properly circulate. This is more commonly seen in hot-flash environments with concurrent qi stagnation and qi deficiency.

When indicated, SP10 is a very easy point to add to any combination. It can be used in conjunction with other points along the spleen channel. SP1 and LR1 can be added for especially problematic issues of heavy and continual periods due to qi deficiency, stagnation, or heat repletion.

PC3 (QUZE) 曲泽

PC3 is an effective point for treating hot flashes. It is a wonderful alternative point to use when PC6 or PC8 are too sensitive for patients. I utilize this point in patients with concurrent hot flashes and digestive issues.

PC3 is especially effective at resolving heat and stagnation due to digestive issues. When qi is knotted in the stomach, qi cannot descend and in turn generates heat and rebels upwards. The stomach sits on the other side of the diaphragm directly below the heart. Stomach heat rises and harasses the heart fire.

PC6 is the premier acupoint on the body for resolving stomach qi, but PC3 is more effective for chronic stagnation and heat repletion conditions, especially those due to poor dietary habits or being exposed to unsanitary food conditions.

PC3 can be very sensitive when improperly needled. The elbow is a network rich in blood vessels and nerves. It is necessary to needle into the soft tissues on the ulnar side of the bicep tendon with the patient's arm slightly bent.

Calming the Shen

It is necessary to use sedation acupuncture points for some menopausal-transition patients. These patients have heightened conditions of hyperactive yang qi, stagnation, heat repletion, chronic yin, or blood depletion that have severely affected the heart spirit.

These patients may not even start out by seeking help for hot flashes. Their primary concern may be insomnia or anxiety that has risen dramatically during menopausal transition. In some cases, it will not only be necessary to clear fire, subdue yang qi, regulate qi, and nourish deficiency; it will also be necessary to specifically sedate and calm the shen.

Several effective spirit calming points have already been described, including DU20, DU24, HT7, HT8, PC8, LI4, and LR3. The following points can be added to any prescription for further sedative purposes.

KI1 (YONGQUAN) 涌泉

KI1 is arguably the best point on the body to sedate and calm the spirit. Located on the sole of the foot, it has the innate ability to ground the spirit and function as a recharging station.

This point also carries a powerful descending and clearing action. As the lowest point on the body, needling KI1 is like punching a hole in the bottom of a barrel to allow the contents to drain out. It is able to clear heart and liver fire and anchor hyperactive yang qi.

KI1 is also able to reestablish the water and fire balance between the kidney and heart. KI1 is called "rushing spring." Needling KI1 generates kidney water, which rushes up from the spring and quells the heart fire. Along with acupuncture, I like to use a TDP (Teding Diancibo Pu) lamp at this point to enhance its functionality.

KI1 on the sole of the foot is the mirror image of PC8 on the palm of the hand. Together, they are a powerful sedation combination. They are well-known points in qi gong practice. While KI1 connects the body to the ground, PC8 reaches up and connects the body to the heavens.

KI1 can be used for intractable hot flashes, anxiety, and insomnia. It is a challenging point to needle and has the same needling principles as PC8 and HT8. The skin can be very sensitive at KI1 and it takes a special touch. Insertion must penetrate deep enough as to not get caught up in the skin surface. If this happens, it will create sharpness and pain. It will become even more intense if the practitioner continues by trying to push the needle through the superficial layers.

The key to successful KI1 insertion is to gently press into the tissues as the needle is firmly inserted without hesitation. Once the needle tip is through the superficial skin layer, there is less discomfort. Most patients are fine and without discomfort once the needle reaches the desired depth and qi sensation is achieved.

Patients who have KI1 needled regularly become accustomed to it and have very few issues. It is good practice to prepare the patient by explaining that this point may elicit a quick sting.

GB13 (BENSHEN) 本神 AND SISHENCONG (M-HN-1) 四神聪

GB13 and Sishencong function to calm the spirit. They can be added to DU20 and DU24 for treating patients with difficult spirit conditions, such as increased anxiety and insomnia during menopausal transition. When the term shen is noted in an acupuncture point's name, it reveals the point's ability to treat the spirit. GB13, DU24, and Sishencong (san shen xue "three shen points" 三神穴) all have shen in their name and together, they create an excellent sedation point combination. Sishencong also has the ability to raise the yang qi to treat mental fatigue and poor concentration commonly seen in menopausal-transition patients.

YINTANG (M-HN-3) "HALL OF IMPRESSION" 印堂

Yintang has a strong sedating function and is used to calm the spirit and enhance clarity. It can be included with any acupuncture treatment to address stress or confusion. I prefer to use this point for patients who have difficulty with relaxation or resolution issues.

Qi and Blood Regulation

Various stagnations within the body contribute to and exacerbate the hot-flash environment. It is often necessary to address them by adding additional points to a hot-flash prescription.

Habitual stagnations typically develop over longer periods of time. They are often the result of qi and blood or yin and yang imbalances stemming from menstrual-cycle abnormalities, stress and emotional instabilities, dietary irregularities, and other various unsuitable lifestyle traits. It is essential to review the patient health intake forms and notes to look for signs of stagnation. The goal is to resolve stagnation and return the health environment to homeostasis with additional stagnation resolving acupuncture points.

GB34 (YANGLINGQUAN) 阳陵泉 AND SJ6 (ZHIGOU) 支沟

The GB34 and SJ6 combination has a strong therapeutic action, addressing and relieving difficult and chronic qi stagnation.

Common qi stagnation situations routinely resolve without intervention. When qi stagnation becomes problematic, acupuncture and herbal formulas can easily remedy the condition. In some women, however, stagnations become habitual and problematic to resolve. As agitators return over and over again, like the tides of the ocean, the patient can no longer release qi and the pattern becomes stuck.

GB34 and SJ6 are effective for relieving long-standing qi depression that blocks smooth qi and blood flow within the zangfu organs. Symptoms can include pain and soreness along the liver and gallbladder channels, tightness through the chest, heart palpitations, difficulty breathing, diaphragm and abdominal tension, digestion disruption, trouble with concentration, headaches, sensory organ issues, depression, irritability, and anxiety. Long-standing qi depression will agitate heart fire, further affecting menopausal-transition symptoms like sleep disruption, emotional instability, and hot flashes.

ST36 (ZUSANLI) 足三里, ST37 (SHANGJUXU) 上巨虚, AND ST39 (XIAJUXU) 下巨虚

It is essential to address any digestive issue throughout menopausal transition to allow the body to regenerate and find its new balance.

Difficulties can appear anywhere along the digestive tract. In Chinese medicine, digestive issues typically happen within the upper abdomen where the stomach resides, or within the lower abdomen where the large and small intestines reside.

Problems of excess, deficiency, stagnation, heat, and cold are common and are due to dietary and lifestyle issues. Digestive difficulties become heightened during menopausal transition. Both acute and chronic digestive issues need to be addressed, not only to allow for the healthy production of qi and blood, but also to relieve the taxation on the body.

ST36 along with ST30 are the transporting points for the sea of water and grains. ST37 and ST39 along with BL11 are the transporting points for the sea of blood and the chong mai.

I like to call this point combination the "three sea points." My professor, Dr. Qiu Hua Shan, first introduced me to this combination. She revealed this combination to me for resolving problematic digestive issues. It consists of the stomach, large intestine, and small intestine he-sea/lower he-sea points for the three major digestive fu organs. The he-sea points are traditionally used for treating fu organ disorders. The fu organs are the digestive organs.

These three points are perfectly aligned along the stomach channel and spaced three cun or inches apart in consecutive order. I alternatively consider them as the "three cun points." It is easy to administer this point combination to patients with a history of irregular and problematic digestive issues.

What makes these points even more important for treating hot flashes is the sea of blood and the chong mai connection. Tonifying the sea of blood nourishes the heart and controls the upward surging tendency of the chong mai, thus quelling hot flashes.

ST40 (FENGLONG) 丰隆

It is worth considering ST40 for its strong action of relieving chronic qi and phlegm stagnation. Long-standing stagnation issues, whether due to excess or deficiency, have the tendency for phlegm to develop. ST40 has long been considered the primary acupuncture point on the body for resolving phlegm due to any pattern.

ST40 has a dual function of resolving qi and phlegm stagnation. This point can be added to any acupuncture prescription when phlegm is involved. ST40 should be utilized for problematic patients that don't respond to traditional acupuncture therapeutic methods. Chinese medicine considers all stubborn and chronic conditions a result of phlegm.

LR13 (ZHANGMEN) 章门

LR13 is the spleen front-mu point, zang organs hui-influential point, and a liver and gallbladder channels crossing point. It is very effective at resolving both emotional and digestive stagnation issues with its ability to harmonize the spleen and liver.

Experienced practitioners know that liver-spleen disharmony is quite common in the clinic. It is the result of stress, dietary irregularities, and lifestyle choices. LR13 is located above the liver on the right and the spleen on the left side of the upper abdomen.

LR13 is extremely effective at soothing stubborn liver qi stagnation, especially by opening up the diaphragm. Once qi stagnation is released, qi and blood circulation is restored, and nourishment can once again be supplied to the heart, thus treating hot flashes and other meno-pausal-transition symptoms. I have found LR13 to be one of the most effective points and have used it extensively in my clinical practice.

LU6 (KONGZUI) 孔最

LU6 is the xi-cleft point on the lung channel, giving it a strong function of dispersing and descending lung qi. It is a point well-suited to men-opausal-transition patients who have tendencies for chest exuberance, often due to an excess deficiency pattern. LU6 has a strong qi function and it is necessary to use it with caution in patients with sea of qi, yin, or blood deficiency patterns.

> **Plum pit qi case study:** A 51-year-old female patient presented with moderate nighttime-only hot flashes with little night sweat-ing. Accompanying symptoms included atrial fibrillation and heart palpitations that were better in the morning and worse in the evening, constipation, gas, bloating, difficulty in falling asleep, and high stress and anxiety due to the recent death of her parents. The patient cleaned houses for a living and was exposed to clean-ing chemicals. She rested very little during her workday. She was pleasant and jovial. Her pulse was deep, slippery, and forceless. Her tongue was puffy and dry with a thick white coating.
>
> The original diagnosis was spleen qi and kidney essence defi-ciency with liver and stomach qi stagnation. Chronic qi stagnation generates fire and consumes qi and blood while blocking body fluids movement. Since the patient did not want to take herbs, I used a general hot-flash deficiency acupuncture prescription. After four treatments, there were fewer palpitations and less anxiety and stress, with a 15–20% improvement in hot flashes. Since there was no change in her constipation, I included SJ6 and GB34. After two more sessions, the palpitations and hot flashes improved another 5–10%.
>
> Upon reevaluation, I noticed the patient kept clearing her throat. I changed the acupuncture prescription to treat plum pit qi derived from qi stagnation and phlegm. I used the following prescription: DU20, DU24, LU7, KI6, ST9, LU1, RN22, RN12,

RN6, RN4, LR13, LR5, ST40, SP4, PC6, HT7, SJ6, KI3. After one treatment, the palpitations were gone, hot flashes were minimal, sleep was good, constipation and stress were relieved, and throat clearing was better.

My conclusion is that once the throat qi was opened, the liver soothed, and the stomach qi descended; everything fitted into place. This allowed the spleen and kidney to strengthen their roles and reestablish communication with the heart. This calmed the heart shen because there was no longer fire as a result of qi stagnation harassing the shen. The patient came in for three more treatments (ten in total) and felt her recovery was satisfactory.

Chest and Abdominal Points

Simple reasoning supports adding local acupuncture points for the chest and abdomen to stimulate the zangfu organs that reside within. The concept uses local points to treat local problems.

Local chest and upper and lower abdominal points along the ren, kidney, stomach, spleen, gallbladder, and liver channels can be utilized to address problems. Chest and abdominal points are necessary to treat both excess and deficiency patterns and should be added for local qi stagnation and digestive imbalances.

This discussion is intended only as an introduction. There are too many chest and abdominal acupuncture points to cover in this book. A few primary acupoints are highlighted. Clinicians will find it relatively easy to select additional acupoints to address specific local issues.

RN17 (SHANZHONG) 膻中

RN17 is located in the center of the chest in front of the heart and lungs. It is the front-mu point of the pericardium and the hui-influential point for qi, and is known as the sea of qi. RN17 functions to reestablish qi and blood circulation throughout the chest region. Not only is it able to gather qi and blood to the area when it is deficient, it can also descend qi and blood when it is in excess. Proper balance of the heart and lung is essential to good health in general, and RN17 is an effective point for treating imbalances that develop during menopausal transition.

LU1 (ZHONGFU) 中府

LU1 is the front-mu point of the lung and is perhaps the most powerful point for stimulating the lung qi. Stimulating lung qi promotes the lung-kidney connection. It is also the crossing point of the lung and spleen channels and has the function of generating qi. LU1 and RN17 are a good combination to open the flow of qi in the chest to relax chest tightness, relieve shallow breathing, and lessen exuberance in the heart.

RN14 (JUQUE) 巨阙

RN14 can be added along the top of the upper abdomen to resolve diaphragm stagnation. Releasing the diaphragm reestablishes qi communication between the lung and kidney.

RN14 is the front-mu point of the heart. Its wide array of functions in resolving excess and deficiency heart patterns makes it an effective point to add during menopausal transition. It is useful in treating symptoms such as anxiety, palpitations, insomnia, and hot flashes.

RN10 (XIAWAN) 下脘 AND RN12 (ZHONGWAN) 中脘

RN10 and RN12 are very effective points for acute and chronic stomach issues, such as problems with bloating, pain, stomach qi rebellion, and stomach heat issues.

Located in the center of the upper abdomen, the front-mu point of the stomach and the hui-influential point for the fu organs, RN12 is a versatile point for any stomach digestive disorder. However, I have found RN10 to have a stronger effect for treating excess, while RN12 is better suited to resolving deficient patterns. This is the result of the location of RN12 in front of and at the same level as the spleen and stomach, which are in charge of generating post-heaven qi. I find the center of the abdomen to be nourishing in nature.

RN9 (SHUIFEN) 水分

RN9 is widely utilized to treat the accumulation of body fluids. Its name, Shuifen, means "water divide," illustrating its action of transforming fluids. RN9 is positioned in front of the small intestine, which controls this function.

Body fluids typically gather when kidney, spleen, and lung yang qi are weak and can no longer transform and transport the fluids. Located just above the umbilicus at the body midline center, RN9 is able to reestablish proper separation performed by the small intestine and the proper dispersal of the body fluids by the lung, spleen, and kidney. If a patient has issues of water accumulation, swelling, or edema, adding RN9 can address this situation.

ST25 (TIANSHU) 天枢, SP15 (DAHENG) 大横, AND GB26 (DAIMAI) 带脉

ST25, SP15, and GB26 are all located along the midline, outwards from the umbilicus (RN8). These points help regulate the ascending and descending qi and blood flow along the abdominal channels and are used for stimulating zangfu organ and digestive issues due to deficiency and stagnation.

ST30 (QICHONG) 气冲

Qichong means rushing qi. ST30 is a meeting point of the stomach channel and the chong mai. The character for chong in qichong is identical to that of the chong mai. This is no coincidence. ST30's connection to the chong mai results in two important menopausal transition applications.

First, it regulates qi and blood in the uterus and lower abdomen. This is particularly useful during early menopausal transition when qi and blood flow becomes more erratic as the chong mai slowly dries up.

Second, ST30 controls upward rushing qi along the channel. Chong mai, stomach, and liver qi all have a natural ascending nature. This nature can be accentuated in an imbalanced hot-flash environment where deficiency is unable to control excess. This ascending qi can bring ministerial fire along with it, harassing the heart fire. This is a common hot-flash pattern.

ST9 (RENYING) 人迎

Located on the neck in front of the thyroid gland, ST9 is perhaps the most useful point in aiding qi and blood circulation to the head and brain. In Western medical practice, it is necessary to maintain proper nourishment and hormone circulation to and from the brain to help regulate the HPO axis. In Chinese medicine, ST9 is a window-of-heaven point that establishes and maintains proper qi and blood flow to and from the head.

In theory, ST9 could be used for all menopausal patients. However, it is a technically challenging and potentially dangerous acupoint to needle. Once proficiency has been established, it is not very difficult to use ST9 in the clinic, but extra caution is warranted.

Back Acupuncture Treatments

Back-shu acupuncture points are generally suggested for treating most zangfu organ patterns in Chinese-medicine acupuncture practice. For example, BL15 (heart) and BL23 (kidney) are traditionally used for treating menopausal-transition symptoms due to heart and kidney yin deficiency.

Most clinical practitioners treat only one side of the patient per treatment. Treating the front is usually the default. Some practitioners will alternate the front and back from treatment to treatment, especially if the patient is coming in for multiple treatments per week. Unless the patient is seeking neck, spine, low back, or hip treatment, it is less likely that many practitioners would adopt back treatments.

Some patients will respond better to treatments on one side than the other. This is somewhat similar to some patients responding better to treatments during the morning or evening time. It may not be possible to establish a reason for the difference. One consideration might be that if a patient requires more yin stimulation perhaps treating the front would be preferred, while a patient that requires more yang stimulation or regulation may respond better to back treatment.

The bladder and du channels located on the back are yang in nature. This does not mean that points along these channels are only used to stimulate yang. Acupuncture study suggests the back-shu points of the zangfu organs are able to drain repletion and supplement deficiency. Theoretically, anyone could needle the back zang-organ shu points to treat menopausal transition. But are back treatments as effective as front treatments? The short answer is—yes.

Back-Shu Points

My clinical experience suggests that only three back-shu points are needed. This is based on which organs are excessive or deficient in the hot-flash environment. I generally select the points based on axis, trajectories, and triads diagnosis.

For general deficiency, it is necessary to stimulate the lung, spleen, and kidney by needling BL13, BL20, and BL23.

For water and fire, yin and yang imbalance, it is necessary to regulate the kidney, liver, and heart by needling BL15, BL18, and BL23.

For nourishing qi and blood, it is necessary to stimulate the kidney, spleen, and heart by needling BL15, BL20, and BL23.

For qi and blood circulation, it is necessary to stimulate the kidney, lung, and heart by needling BL13, BL15, and BL23.

For relative excess patterns, it is necessary to clear the liver, spleen, and heart by needling BL15, BL18, and BL20.

For relative deficiency patterns, it is necessary to nourish the kidney, liver, and spleen by needling BL18, BL20, and BL23.

Du-Mai Points

The selection of du-mai points along the spine is based on location and function. In general, they have powerful actions, especially on yang qi and the nervous system. Two major du-mai points to consider are DU14 and DU4.

DU14 (DAZHUI) 大椎

DU14 is the meeting point of all six yang channels. It is a yang qi beacon. DU14 is a primary point for clearing many types of heat, including heart fire.

DU14 is listed as a primary acupuncture point for treating tidal heat effusion of any pattern. It is also used to regulate the ying and wei qi and is indicated for treating sweating disorders, including night sweating. This dual action makes DU14 a useful point in treating menopausal-transition patients.

DU4 (MINGMEN) 命门

DU4 has the ability to both excite yang qi and clear heat from the zangfu organs. In some hot-flash patients, it is necessary to stoke yang qi within the mingmen to generate new and fresh yin. In other patients, it is essential to drain excess fire. DU4 has the powerful ability to simultaneously supplement yin and clear yang. This dual action makes it a prominent point for treating hot flashes and menopausal transition.

Neck Points

Acupuncture points on the back of the neck are extremely useful in treating hot flashes in menopausal transition. DU16, BL10, and GB20 are located on a horizontal line across the base of the occiput. Together, they produce results similar to ST9, improving qi and blood circulation to the head and brain. The difference is ST9 has a yin function and works on the qi and blood, whereas DU16, BL10, and GB20 have a yang function and work to regulate yin and yang within the brain. Together, these four points maintain neurotransmission and balance the HPO axis.

Supporting Back Points

Relatively few supporting acupuncture points along the extremities are needed to support back treatments. Points along the yin channels are helpful for enhancing yin nourishing functions, while points along the taiyang and shaoyang channels are helpful for enhancing yang regulating functions.

Here are three effective and efficient two-point combination additions: KI3 and BL60 to balance yin and yang; SP6 and HT7 to enhance qi and blood; GB34 and PC6 to regulate qi.

Auricular Acupuncture

Women have very busy lives with work, family, relationship, and social responsibilities. This can make it challenging to commit both precious time and finances to self-care and well-being. Acupuncture treatments two or three times per week is just out of the question for many patients, but reducing this to one acupuncture treatment per week may produce effects more slowly and may be less effective for some patients.

Auricular seed therapy, in conjunction with body acupuncture, is a valuable treatment option. Practitioners can certainly needle auricular points during clinic treatments instead of using seed therapy. The use of the auricular seed therapy, however, enhances the benefits and effectiveness of body acupuncture over a longer period of time and until the next treatment. This allows for a steady and gradual increase in effectiveness rather than the up-and-down progress that can occur when using acupuncture alone. Patients will notice the positive results with the addition of the auricular option.

Auricular acupuncture in itself is a vast and independent therapeutic system. Much like acupuncture and herbal medicine, there are many points, combinations, and approaches. Here is a list of clinically effective auricular points: Shenmen 神门, Uterus 子宫, Kidney 肾, Heart 心, Liver 肝, Spleen 脾, Pituitary 脑垂体, Sympathetic 交感, Endocrine 内分泌, Neurasthenia 神经衰弱点.

Shenmen is widely recognized and one of the most commonly used ear acupuncture points. Its main function is to tranquilize the mind, and it helps with the treatment of nervous and cardiovascular system disorders. Shenmen allows these systems to relax and reestablish balance. For menopausal-transition patients, it is ideal for treating hot flashes, insomnia, and anxiety.

The uterus point is added to any treatment to help regulate menstrual irregularities and abnormal bleeding commonly seen during early menopausal transition. It helps treat heavy or irregular periods, spotting, long or constant bleeding, and associated disorders such as fibroids, polyps, cysts, and endometriosis.

The kidney ear point functions to strengthen the zangfu aspects of the kidney organ. It nourishes essence and the sea of marrow, and regulates the HPO axis. The kidney is able to treat symptoms stemming from neurological, gynecological, and urogenital disorders.

The heart ear point functions to nourish and regulate the zangfu aspects of the heart. In conjunction with the kidney, it balances the water and fire, yin and yang between the two organs. The heart is essential in treating hot flashes, insomnia, and anxiety.

The liver and spleen are adjunctive points. Together, they function to bring support and balance back to the yin and yang and zangfu organs. They are well-suited to a wide variety of menopausal-transition symptoms.

The pituitary point has a strong effect on the regulation of the HPO axis and endocrine system. It is recommended for treating mood swings and emotional issues, as well as sleep difficulties.

The sympathetic point is used for numerous diseases related to autonomic nervous system dysfunction. It has a special ability to treat anxiety, palpitations, sweating, and hot flashes.

The endocrine point harmonizes endocrine-system function. For menopausal-transition patients, it is ideal for regulating the natural disruption in the HPO axis.

The neurasthenia point is a great addition for the menopausal-transition patient with insomnia. It treats sleeping issues including the inability to fall asleep, light sleep, and waking at night.

Both acupuncture and auricular seed therapy can be used on every patient. After an acupuncture session, auricular seeds are applied to one ear after properly locating the most tender area of each point. Choose the best points based on the need of the patient. Five to six points is sufficient in most cases.

Seeds are retained for an average of five to seven days. Seed therapy loses its therapeutic strength over time. Patients should be taught how to press each seed to induce qi sensation five times per day. The patient can remove any seeds that are uncomfortable. Seed therapy should alternate from one side to the other each week to maintain fresh stimulation of the auricular points.

Acupuncture and Hot Flashes Scientific Research

Acupuncture exists because it's effective. Current research has produced an overwhelming body of data supporting the efficacy of acupuncture in treating problems in the body's complex network of systems. The Evidence Based Acupuncture Group is an excellent resource and provides up-to-date information.

A pressing concern is the lack of randomized controlled trials (RCTs). Acupuncture RCTs have many logistical difficulties, including funding, size, location, and training in obtaining reliable data. One major challenge is the strong placebo effect that acupuncture transmits (Avis and Coeytaux 2010). This makes setting up double-blind studies virtually impossible. Sham procedures serving the placebo role are difficult to design… and there is no way to have a skilled acupuncturist not know if they are applying the sham or real acupuncture treatment. Nonetheless, it is possible to collect clinical evidence that strongly supports the efficacy of acupuncture in general.

More specifically, clinical evidence confirms the efficacy of acupuncture in treating hot flashes (Borud *et al.* 2009). One large meta-analysis considered the data from 104 studies and "confirms that acupuncture improves hot flash frequency and severity, menopause-related symptoms, and quality of life (in the vasomotor domain) in women experiencing natural menopause" (Chiu *et al.* 2015, p.234).

Acupuncture is useful for treating menopause-related problems, and increased understanding and training can make it even more effective. There is still much to be learned. For example, researchers are working to identify bio-markers that can predict things like how severe hot flashes are likely to be and how effective acupuncture will be in treating them (Thurston and Joffe 2011; Ziv-Gal *et al.* 2017).

Quantity and Duration of Treatments

Hot flashes do respond to acupuncture, but that response is highly variable in individuals. For many treatments, the period of time required to produce satisfactory results will vary. Most acupuncture studies administer on average 6–20 treatments over a few weeks to a few months. Results vary from patient to patient (Avis *et al.* 2017). One study reports:

> the maximal reduction in hot flashes occurred at week 7, which corresponds to a median of eight acupuncture treatments. After week 8,

> the median cumulative number of treatments continued to increase
> to a median of 18 at week 26, whereas the percent change in VMS
> frequency did not. (Avis *et al.* 2016, p.629)

Fewer treatments result in less efficacy, while results from prolonged
treatments level off.

Once efficacy is achieved and treatments taper off, hot flashes do
sometimes return. For the duration of hot flashes, "with the average
being 6 months to 2 years with possibility as long as 10.2 years" (Freeman *et al.* 2011), it may be necessary to follow active treatment with
a series of routine maintenance treatments for satisfactory control of
hot flashes. Every woman's body will respond differently. Some may
need maintenance treatments every week, every two weeks, once
per month, or merely once every quarter. Some will not require any
additional treatments.

Chinese-Medicine Pattern Differentiation and Diagnosis

Chinese-medicine pattern differentiation and diagnosis is sometimes
used in acupuncture research, and the description of the protocol
suggests how ongoing diagnosis may result in improved results by
adjusting acupuncture treatment:

> TCM diagnoses were reassessed (and changed, if indicated) at each
> subsequent treatment session. Study acupuncturists were permitted to
> change acupuncture point selection and other aspects of treatment if
> clinically indicated at each treatment session. (Avis *et al.* 2017, p.173)

A thorough and reasoned diagnosis is a good predictor of how well a
hot-flash case will respond to acupuncture treatment, and treatment
may be improved if the clinician is able to modify treatments based on
improved understanding of underlying conditions.

I have been diagnosing the hot-flash environment in women for
many years, and I still find it can be challenging. Pattern differentiation
and diagnosis can sometimes be unreliable and misleading. General
theories can only go so far when faced with the infinite variations
within individuals. If the practitioner does not have significant

hot-flash experience, they may find their effectiveness limited, requiring much deeper understanding of Chinese-medicine theory.

Using Chinese-medicine pattern differentiation and diagnosis for choosing an appropriate effective acupuncture prescription in scientific research has another limitation. There is significant variation in how different practitioners diagnose the hot-flash environment and select acupuncture prescriptions. The research shows overall efficacy of acupuncture, but without being able to standardize diagnosis, it is difficult to draw more detailed conclusions.

How Can We Improve Clinical Acupuncture Efficacy in Treating Hot Flashes?

The hot-flash environment is a short list of root patterns with a longer list of accompanying subsequent branch (symptomatic) patterns. The basic symptom, of course, is heat or fire. Most practitioners inadvertently focus on this symptom and fail to see the root pattern. Common root patterns include yang rising with yin deficiency, qi and blood deficiency, heat repletion, and chronic stagnation.

Most hot-flash patterns are a combination of excess, deficiency, and stagnation. Every hot-flash environment is unique in that regard and will respond best to a specific acupuncture prescription: supplementation, draining, or regulation.

Individualized Versus Standardized Acupuncture-Point Prescriptions

There are pros and cons to having individualized and standardized acupuncture-point prescriptions to treat hot flashes. Individuated care developed by the acupuncturist and tailored to the patient will most closely represent her unique experience in the world. On the other hand, a series of standardized prescriptions can target specific issues and bio-markers and take a lot of guesswork out of the clinic, simplifying the process and making it possible for people with less knowledge, training, and experience to find some success in treating hot flashes. Standardized prescriptions also allow for more controlled research. Although both have their positives, many acupuncturists and Chinese-medicine practitioners may choose to continue providing treatment based on individual assessment.

Individualized Points

Acupuncture-point prescription is a concern in acupuncture research. Many studies allow the acupuncturist to use Chinese-medicine pattern differentiation and diagnosis and then choose an acupuncture-point prescription accordingly. This presents issues based on non-standardized diagnosis and variations in prescriptions from one acupuncturist to the next.

Based on learning experiences and style of practice, it is common to find significant variation in diagnosis and treatment among practitioners. Research results are strongly affected by these variables and thus hard to interpret. One hot-flash case might theoretically be diagnosed and treated quite differently by two practitioners. One may be effective and one ineffective, but this result, though reported, cannot differentiate if the efficacy or lack of it was based on the diagnosis, the prescription, or the skill of the practitioner. There are just so many variables from one practitioner to the next, based on training, belief, and ability to diagnose, that it is difficult to draw any meaningful conclusions from reported results.

This style of study allows for different acupuncture prescriptions to be used on different patients who may have had the same diagnosis. Research results are showing that acupuncture may be effective in treating hot flashes, but for the most part, this research doesn't have the scientific rigor to help find improvements for the treatment of hot flashes.

While it has some merit, non-standardized research has severe limitations. There are no set parameters. It is common knowledge that certain acupuncture points, based on Chinese medicine and scientific evidence, have greater impact on the organs, brain, and overall system, than do other points. Certainly, research proving that acupuncture treats hot flashes is worthwhile. Research suggests that many women will benefit, even if it is based on the routine application of standard acupuncture.

Standardized Points

Research based on standardized sets of points helps to establish the general effectiveness of these points. The chosen point prescription typically utilizes a set of strong and commonly used acupoints. This research advances our knowledge because it demonstrates how well a particular prescription works. Prescriptions like this can be easily employed in any clinical setting. This removes guesswork from the equation and the need to differentiate between patients. This is especially good for Western practitioners of acupuncture that do not utilize Chinese-medicine pattern differentiation and diagnosis.

A significant drawback to using a generalized prescription is that certain patients will not respond as well, if at all, to the chosen set of points. This supports the creation of a series of standardized hot-flash acupuncture prescriptions. The ideal situation in acupuncture research is to discover which acupuncture points work to their greatest strengths in conjunction with other acupoints to form an eloquent acupuncture-point prescription to treat one specific hot-flash pattern.

The ideal outcome of research would be the identification of certain acupuncture points or prescriptions that turn hot flashes off like a light switch. But until that perfect solution is found, we will continue to provide what we know is an effective and comparatively inexpensive treatment to alleviate the severity of hot flashes for many women.

I hypothesize that acupuncture on its own has the potential to reach an overall 75% effectiveness rate in treating hot flashes. Curative rates could potentially reach around 90% with the correct additions of Chinese herbal formulas, vitamins and supplements, and productive lifestyle changes including things like diet, hydration, meditation, yoga (Ee *et al.* 2017), walking, light exercise, proper rest, and stress modifiers.

Chapter 7

Treating Hot Flashes with Chinese Herbal Medicine

Treatment Principles

It is difficult to clear fire by only nourishing water. It is difficult to replenish water by only clearing fire. To balance fire and water, it is imperative to treat both at the same time. But this way of thinking will not suffice. It is essential to address the root issue causing the fire and water imbalance.

The hot flash is a burst of qi manifesting as heat. Treating hot flashes is not simply about nourishing yin or clearing fire. Truly and effectively healing the hot-flash environment requires the heat, repletion, stagnation, and deficiency to be addressed.

Practitioners need to pose the following questions: Is there heat? Is it one of excess or deficiency? Is it being generated from a repletion, stagnation, or deficiency pattern? Is it systemic or stemming from any particular organ(s)? Is there damp-phlegm, qi stagnation, blood stasis, or cold or heat repletion involved? Are qi and blood, yin and yang, body fluids and essence healthy or deficient? Each patient has a distinct situation. Answering these questions will guide us to the most suitable herbal formula for remedying the hot-flash environment.

Hot-flash herbal formula composition will be based on the following principles.

- Clearing heat

- Balancing yin and yang

- Regulating qi

- Nourishing qi and blood, yin and yang

- Calming the shen.

It's not mandatory to include all five components or to address them in any particular order. The beauty of herbal medicine is the ability to combine the right percentages of each group to target the specific needs of the patient. In fact, when we look at many of the formulas to treat hot flashes, many of them are similar in nature and utilize many of the same herbs but in different dosages and strengths.

Hot-Flash Herbal Formulas

The following sections contain descriptions and commentary on the primary Chinese herbal formulas for treating the hot-flash environment. Formulas for treating excess heat conditions are presented first, followed by those that address repletion and stagnation patterns, those that address deficiency conditions, and finally calming the spirit formulas.

It is not possible to highlight every possible formula for treating hot flashes. You may also have developed a different approach and use different formulas, perhaps utilizing modern formulas based on your research and personal experience. The strength of Chinese medicine is, at its core, that we are all practicing the same medicine based on the same theories. Similar formulas will have similar effects even though we may be using different herbal prescriptions and strategies.

Most of the formulas are found in general use throughout Chinese medicine. I have not included the herbal weights and dosages. Most patent formulas adhere to the original prescription. Please refer to reference manuals for specific questions regarding herbs, formulas, and dosages. When preparing your own herbal formulas, please adhere to the recommended dosages from the textbooks or modify appropriately.

Patent Herbal Formulas

Many acupuncturists and Chinese-medicine practitioners are limited to only being able to use patent formulas. Patent formulas are premade herbal formulas that come in pill, tablet, or capsule form. Other practitioners have an herbal dispensary of whole or powdered herbs and formulas. These practitioners can fully utilize Chinese herbal medicine by providing precise formulas tailored to the individual needs of their patients. Most of the listed herbal formulas are available in patent formulas. A few may be more difficult to obtain in premade form.

For practitioners using patent formulas who are unable to prepare individualized formulas, it is safe and often effective to prescribe two or more patent formulas together for a patient. For instance, you can theoretically use a deficiency formula along with a qi stagnation, heat clearing, or shen sedation formula. Lastly, for those practitioners who cannot or do not use herbal formulas, this may not be of great concern. I treat most of my hot-flash patients without using herbs and have great success.

STRENGTH AND COST

Not all patent formulas are the same. Depending on the manufacturer, some may be stronger or weaker than others. This is often reflected in the price. An inexpensive formula may be weaker in nature, meaning more is required to achieve the same effect as its more expensive counterpart.

SAFETY

Most reputable companies have adopted international testing and safety standards to ensure their herbs and formulas are safe for medical treatment. Be sure to use reputable companies. Resources on Chinese herbal companies and manufacturers can be easily located.

MODIFICATIONS

Some manufacturers modify their patent formulas. This can be beneficial in some respects because they will add the necessary herbs to a traditional formula to make it more effective. By adding additional herbs, they are able to target common problems. As a practitioner, the downside to these brands is more is not necessarily better. You end up prescribing additional herbs when the traditional formula would be preferred. I use both traditional patent formulas and modified formulas from multiple companies. Through clinical observation, I've observed which modifications have better therapeutic effects in some patients and when the traditional formula is more appropriate.

Above all, it is important to maintain diagnostic accuracy whether using acupuncture in conjunction with herbs or just herbs on their own. Herbal medicine needs to be specific to the patient. It is less forgiving than acupuncture when dealing with excesses and deficiencies. The tongue and pulse, along with careful diagnosis, should give you an accurate pattern to find the most appropriate formula for the patient.

Heat Clearing Herbs

Clearing heat is a generalized term and incorporates the elimination of pathogenic warmth, heat, and fire with various methods. One way to clear heat is to use cold medicinals: "When heat is treated with cold, cold drugs are employed to treat heat illness" (Unschuld and Tessenow 2011, p.352).

Heat enters and manifests in the body in several ways, including heat from external invasion of pathogenic factors, febrile disease, heat accumulation in the channels and zangfu organs, heat in the nutritive and blood levels, damp-heat accumulation, yin fire, heat from deficiency, and so on. Depending on the severity and location, heat in the body presents in different ways and exhibits with different and unique symptoms.

Herbs that clear heat are categorized based on their properties and the type of heat they treat. In modern medicine, many heat clearing herbs are used for their antipyretic, anti-inflammatory, and antimicrobial properties.

HEAT CLEARING AND FIRE PURGING HERBS

These herbs are the coldest in nature and are very effective at clearing excess heat and fire pathogenic conditions. Herbs in this category are traditionally used for treating febrile disease with high fever, irritability, thirst, and delirium symptoms.

Heat clearing and fire purging herbs are used for excess heat in the qi level and the yangming level. These herbs often enter the liver, lung, and stomach, which are susceptible to repletion. Common herbs in this category are: shi gao, zhi mu, zhu ye, zhi zi.

Shi gao and zhi mu clear heat, sedate fire, dispel irritability, and relieve thirst. Shi gao is the strongest and is only used in excess conditions, while zhi mu has yin nourishing properties, making it versatile for treating excess and deficiency heat patterns and is why we see zhi mu in many heat clearing formulas. Zhu ye is especially useful for clearing heart fire and for hot flashes due to excess. Zhi zi clears heat from all three jiao. It is an adaptable herb that clears heat and drains damp-heat and is more suitable for excess conditions.

HEAT CLEARING AND DAMPNESS DRYING HERBS

These herbs are bitter, cold, and drying in nature, which can be very harsh on the spleen and stomach. They are used to clear heat, dry dampness, purge fire, and eliminate toxins and are often used with fire draining herbs or heat toxicity herbs.

Heat clearing and dampness drying herbs are particularly useful for damp-heat repletion in the intestines, liver and gallbladder, and lower jiao. Herbs in this category are traditionally used for treating dysentery, urinary disorders, and skin conditions. Common herbs in this category are: huang qin, huang lian, huang bai, long dan cao.

Huang qin, huang lian, and huang bai are known as the "san huang" or "three yellow" herbs. They are very bitter and cold and clear damp-heat and toxic heat from the three jiao: huang qin from the upper jiao (chest); huang lian from the upper and middle jiao (chest and upper abdomen); huang bai from the lower jiao (lower abdomen).

Huang lian is especially effective for sedating fire in the heart and liver, making it useful for hot flashes due to excess. Huang bai can also drain kidney heat and is commonly seen in yin deficiency formulas, along with zhi mu.

Long dan cao is one of the strongest herbs used to sedate liver fire. It should only be used in excess conditions.

HEAT CLEARING AND BLOOD COOLING HERBS

These herbs are cold and bitter, sweet, or salty in nature and clear heat from the deep nutritive (ying) and blood (xue) levels. Some herbs in this category have additional yin nourishing and body fluids generating properties. Heat clearing and blood cooling herbs are used for both excess and deficiency heat patterns, especially those affecting the heart and liver.

Herbs in this category are traditionally used for treating low-grade fever, night sweating, delirium, dry throat, red tongue, and bleeding disorders. Common herbs in this category are: sheng di huang, xuan shen, mu dan pi, chi shao.

Sheng di huang and xuan shen nourish yin and cool blood and are especially effective in treating hot flashes and menopausal-transition symptoms due to deficiency patterns.

Mu dan pi and chi shao clear heat and cool blood. They also invigorate blood and are useful in cases of stagnation and stasis. Mu dan pi is particularly useful for clearing heart fire, while chi shao is particularly useful for clearing liver fire.

HEAT CLEARING AND TOXIN ELIMINATING HERBS

These herbs have a dispersing nature and clear heat and fire toxins. Herbs in this category are traditionally used for treating fevers, sores, inflammation, febrile disease, and viral and other infectious disease. Common herbs in this category are: jin yin hua, lian qiao, da qing ye, ban lan gen.

Jin yin hua and lian qiao clear heat and remove toxins. Da qing ye and ban lan gen eliminate toxins and cool blood.

DEFICIENCY HEAT CLEARING HERBS

These herbs are sweet and cold in nature, making them effective in treating yin deficiency heat patterns. Herbs in this category are traditionally used for treating tidal fever, night sweating, and steaming bone-heat and can be beneficial for treating chronic hot flashes due to yin and blood deficiency.

Deficiency heat clearing herbs enter the kidney and liver channels. Common herbs in this category are: qing hao, di gu pi, yin chai hu, hu huang lian.

Qing hao is the best herb for clearing deficiency heat and the number one herb for treating malaria. Di gu pi clears deficiency heat and cools blood. Yin chai hu and hu huang lian clear deficiency heat and treat tidal fever.

Heat Clearing Herb Cautions

It is appropriate to use the correct herbs and formulas for the correct type of heat. Inappropriate use can exacerbate, extend, or worsen the situation.

Strong heat clearing herbs should be used to treat excess conditions only, while herbs that clear heat and cool blood or clear deficiency heat are more suitable for deficiency conditions.

Heat clearing herbs should be used only when necessary. Overuse can damage yin, body fluids, or the vital qi. Particular heat clearing herbs can damage the spleen and stomach. Once the heat clearing effect is achieved, it is necessary to focus treatment on the underlying root condition so heat does not return.

Chinese Herbal Medicine Safety

Chinese herbal formulas are generally safe when prescribed and appropriately administered by a knowledgeable and skilled licensed provider. There are a few important precautions to consider.

General safety concerns escalate with the use of over-the-counter (OTC) supplements and prescriptions from unlicensed medical practitioners. Regarding menopausal transition and hot flash remedies, there is serious concern about ingredient potency and patients getting ingredients inappropriate to their constitution and overall health.

It is essential for all practitioners to know and understand possible herb-drug interactions. A thorough medical history will include drugs, herbs, and OTC supplements. A responsible professional will consider all of the ingredients and their actions and interactions. The goal is to make sure the patient is getting every appropriate support while not taking anything that is unnecessary or potentially damaging.

Finally, special care must be taken when treating at-risk patients.

Many patients in fragile health who are seeking relief from hot flashes have been treated previously by one or several other medical professionals and may be on multiple medications and supplements. Adding another layer of treatment requires the full picture to be considered. Sometimes the best prescription is to forgo the use of herbal formulas and to focus on the use of acupuncture and lifestyle modifications suggestions.

Traditional Tidal Heat Effusion Herbal Formulas
Yin Deficiency and Blood Depletion Tidal Heat Effusion
Qing Gu San 清骨散 (Cool the Bones Powder) addresses yin deficiency and blood depletion tidal heat effusion manifesting during the afternoon, evening, or nighttime. Accompanying symptoms include waves of low-grade heat that come and go, heat in the palms and soles, heart vexation, insomnia, heart palpitations, night sweating, a red tongue with little coating, and a fine and rapid pulse. This type is most closely related to hot flashes during menopausal transition.

Herbs in the formula: yin chai hu, zhi mu, hu huang lian, di gu pi, qing hao, qin jiao, zhi bie jia, gan cao, dang gui, bai shao.

Yangming Excess Tidal Heat Effusion
Da Cheng Qi Tang 大承气汤 (Major Order Qi Decoction) addresses yangming excess tidal heat effusion, which is different from other tidal heat effusion patterns because it is a constant heat effusion. It is also known as "late-afternoon tidal heat effusion" because the heat becomes increasingly more pronounced at 3–5pm. Accompanying symptoms include streaming sweat on the hands and feet, fullness and pain in the abdomen, constipation, vexation and agitation, a dry and yellow tongue coating, and a deep and forceful pulse.

Herbs in the formula: da huang, mang xiao, zhi shi, hou po.

Spleen and Stomach Qi Deficiency Tidal Heat Effusion

Bu Zhong Yi Qi Tang 补中益气汤 (Tonify the Middle and Augment the Qi Decoction) addresses spleen and stomach qi deficiency tidal heat effusion, which causes morning heat effusion and then abates. Accompanying symptoms include lassitude, weakness of the limbs, spontaneous sweating, white complexion, pale tongue, and a fine or weak pulse.

Herbs in the formula: huang qi, ren shen, bai zhu, zhi gan cao, dang gui, chen pi, sheng ma, chai hu.

Damp-Evil Obstruction Tidal Heat Effusion

Qing Shu Yi Qi Tang 清暑益气汤 (Wang Shi's Clear Summer-Heat and Augment the Qi Decoction) addresses damp-evil obstruction tidal heat effusion due to the external attack of summer-heat. The hot and humid weather of late-summer penetrates and enters the body, impairing the spleen and stomach qi. This form of tidal heat effusion has a gradual recovery with the arrival of autumn. Accompanying symptoms include low-grade fever, thirst, loss of appetite, vexation, agitation, fatigue, weakness, diarrhea, greasy tongue coating, and a fine and rapid pulse.

Herbs in the formula: xi yang shen, shi hu, mai men dong, xi gua pi, he geng, zhu ye, zhi mu, huang lian, gan cao, geng mi.

Blood Stasis Tidal Heat Effusion

Xue Fu Zhu Yu Tang 血俯逐淤汤 (Drive Out Stasis in the Mansion of Blood Decoction) addresses blood stasis tidal heat effusion due to long-standing static blood depression within the body. The stasis gives rise to chronic afternoon tidal heat effusion. Accompanying symptoms include a dry mouth and throat, pain in the body, blue or purplish tongue with possible macules, and a rough and fine pulse.

Herbs in the formula: tao ren, hong hua, chuan xiong, dang gui, sheng di huang, chai hu, zhi ke, jie geng, niu xi, gan cao.

Excess Heat and Fire Prescriptions
Formulas for Hot Flashes

This set of formulas addresses hot flashes due to excess heat and fire patterns. The first two formulas address systemic heat and the following four address heat in the heart, stomach, and liver zangfu organs. It is sometimes necessary to concentrate our treatments on particular organs that are susceptible to repletion heat patterns that can exacerbate the hot-flash environment.

Excess heat and fire patterns develop primarily from repletion and stagnation issues or from deficiency issues. In some cases, this is the result of direct environmental or lifestyle habits. Excess heat and fire patterns need to be dealt with directly no matter what the cause, because heat and fire disrupt yin and yang and consume vital qi.

Some of these formulas are standalone hot-flash formulas to be used in excess hot-flash environments, while other formulas in this group are better suited as add-on formulas. These add-on formulas are particularly useful in helping better understand excess heat patterns, the clearing and supporting functions of the herbs, and how we can adopt their strategies to treating hot flashes.

Excess heat clearing formulas are strong at clearing heat. They are not traditionally recommended for long-term use because they can have detrimental effects on the vital qi.

- Huang Lian Jie Du Tang

- Dang Gui Liu Huang Tang

- Dao Chi San

- Zhu Ye Shi Gao Tang

- Xie Huang San

- Yu Nu Jian

- Long Dan Xie Gan Tang

- Qing Shu Yi Qi Tang.

HUANG LIAN JIE DU TANG

Huang Lian Jie Du Tang 黄连解毒汤 (Coptis Decoction to Relieve Toxicity) is a widely chosen herbal formula for treating hot flashes due to excess heat, whether this is from an external source or is an internally generated heat accumulation.

It is the primary formula for clearing heat and eliminating toxins. Heat repletion starts either in the exterior environment and invades the body or with internal issues that eventually develop into constraint and generate heat. Over time, constrained heat harasses the spirit and consumes the vital qi, including the blood, yin, and yang qi.

Herbs in the formula: huang lian, huang qin, huang bai, zhi zi.

This short-ingredient formula is able to clear heat and purge fire from anywhere in the body and is particularly effective, based on its ability to clear heat from all three jiao.

When heat enters and smolders on the interior or when stagnation and accumulation generate heat or fire, it can aggravate and cause heart fire to flare, causing hot flashes and other menopausal symptoms such as insomnia and emotional issues like anxiety and irritability. Stagnation and heat repletion are primary causes of hot flashes, particularly during the early stages of menopausal transition.

The fire must be drained from the heart. One of the chief herbs in Chinese-medicine materia medica with this action is huang lian. As the primary ingredient, huang lian is able to purge heart and stomach fire. Heart controls fire—draining fire from the heart will lead to the draining of fire in all the organs. Huang qin aids huang lian by purging lung heat in the upper jiao. Huang bai purges the kidney fire in the lower jiao, making it especially useful when ministerial fire/kidney fire builds up in the mingmen. Zhi zi helps purge the fire in the triple jiao through the urine. Zhi zi is effective for draining heat, especially that due to stagnation.

Huang Lian Jie Du Tang is especially useful for patients suffering from hot flashes due to a relatively excess condition, such as accumulated heat repletion. Accompanying symptoms include restlessness, irritability, insomnia, a red tongue and yellow coating, and a forceful and rapid pulse.

Huang Lian Jie Du Tang is especially useful as an anti-inflammatory and antipyretic formula and has a widespread application for treating most types of internal heat and fire symptoms.

Huang Lian Jie Du Tang is a strong formula and should not be used long term without properly supporting the vital qi, since it consists of cooling and bitter herbs that eventually plunder the vital qi. It is smart to eventually treat the heat repletion source if it continues. This formula is traditionally contraindicated in patients with yin deficiency. Clinically, it is helpful in the short term to clear an abundance of heat.

Out of all the excess heat formulas, I use this one the most. It covers a broad range of symptoms and is often an excellent formula to start with to get everything cleared before addressing the root problem. I've used Huang Lian Jie Du Tang successfully multiple times when treating hot-flash patients.

DANG GUI LIU HUANG TANG

Dang Gui Liu Huang Tang 当归六黄汤 (Dang Gui Six Yellow Decoction) treats night sweats and hot flashes in a relatively exuberant yang and deficient yin hot-flash environment. This formula targets raging fire due to deficiency where kidney yin (water) is unable to control the heart yang (fire). Dang Gui Liu Huang Tang is named after the six herbs in the formula that have the Chinese word huang (yellow) in their name.

Herbs in the formula: dang gui, sheng di huang, shu di huang, huang lian, huang qin, huang bai, huang qi.

The first three herbs, dang gui, sheng di huang, and shu di huang, nourish yin to control blazing fire. The second three herbs, huang lian, huang qin, and huang bai, utilize the same powerful heat clearing strategy of Huang Lian Jie Du Tang. The final herb, huang qi, is added to protect the wei qi and prevent excessive sweating. Huang qi also protects stomach qi and further damage to yin and yang from the bitter and cold heat clearing herbs.

Dang Gui Liu Huang Tang is an elegant formula at first glance and theoretically appropriate for treating many types of hot-flash patterns.

Common symptoms include night sweats, tidal fever, irritability, dry stools, a red and dry tongue, and a rapid pulse.

Clinically speaking, it is more effective for treating hot flashes during the early stages of menopausal transition with vigorous fire and where vital qi is still quite intact. It is truly a yin and yang balancing formula. Being a formula to treat excess heat conditions, this is less effective where yin has already been damaged and drained. If this is the case, it is better to adopt formulas that are more suitable for nourishing yin and do not use strong heat clearing herbs.

DAO CHI SAN

Dao Chi San 导赤散 (Guide Out the Red Powder) clears heart fire and nourishes yin. Clinically, it is not well-known for treating hot flashes on its own. It is relevant in this discussion because of its herbal properties that can be added to other formulas.

Herbs in the formula: sheng di huang, zhu ye, mu tong, gan cao.

Sheng di huang enters the heart and kidney to cool blood, nourish yin, generate fluids, and strengthen kidney water to control heart fire. This function makes sheng di huang a versatile herb to be added to many hot-flash formulas. It can easily replace its blood and yin nourishing counterpart shu di huang when it is ideal to nourish blood and clear heat.

Zhu ye alleviates irritability by clearing heat from the heart. It can be added to any formula to quell vigorous heart fire in excess conditions.

Mu tong clears heart fire through the urine. Promoting urination is one of three ways of clearing heat and fire from the body; the other two being inducing sweating and purging heat through the bowels. Promoting urination is a safe and effective way of clearing heat. That is why it is important to encourage hydration. Many heat clearing hot-flash formulas contain herbs that induce diuresis. It is worth noting that one type of mu tong, "guan mu tong," contains aristolochic acid (nephrotoxic) and is quite dangerous if taken long term. For this reason, mu tong is regulated and guan mu tong is difficult to purchase and not used in any patent formulas.

ZHU YE SHI GAO TANG

Zhu Ye Shi Gao Tang 竹叶石膏汤 (Lophatherus and Gypsum Decoction) clears heat, generates fluids, augments the qi, and harmonizes the stomach. This formula is traditionally used for clearing lingering pathogenic heat and relieving fever from febrile disease. Much like Dao Chi San, Zhu Ye Shi Gao Tang is not well-known clinically for directly treating hot flashes. It is relevant in this discussion because of its ability to clear heat from the stomach and direct stomach qi downwards.

Herbs in the formula: zhu ye, shi gao, ren shen, mai men dong, ban xia, zhi gan cao, geng mi.

Zhu ye and shi gao clear lingering stomach heat and heart fire. Shi gao is cold in nature and excellent for clearing heat from the lung and stomach. It is also acrid in nature, allowing it to disperse heat. Therefore, shi gao should not be used long term as its cold nature will injure vital qi or, in cases of deficiency with sweating, its dispersing nature will further injure the heart qi. Ren shen and mai men dong are added to tonify qi and generate fluids to protect from further damage to qi and yin by zhu ye and shi gao. Ban xia is added to help direct qi downwards. This is very important in menopausal transition for patients with stomach heat and stagnation.

XIE HUANG SAN

Xie Huang San 泻黄散 (Drain the Yellow Powder) drains smoldering hidden fire from the interior and from the spleen and stomach. Xie Huang San, much like Dao Chi San, is not a commonly used formula for treating hot flashes. Its effects make it worthy of consideration by a skilled practitioner when treating the hot-flash environment with Chinese herbal medicine.

When there is heat repletion in any zangfu organ, it can transfer and affect other organs. Both the spleen and stomach have a direct connection to the heart via their channels; therefore fire manifesting in either of the two is able to ascend and harass the heart fire.

Herbs in the formula: shi gao, zhi zi, fang feng, huo xiang, gan cao.

Shi gao and zhi zi are used to drain heat from the spleen and stomach and from the three jiao via diuresis. These two herbs are especially effective for abating heart fire, quelling hot flashes, and relieving irritability in excess conditions.

The miraculous addition of fang feng makes this formula noteworthy in its unique ability to clear hidden spleen fire. Formulas utilizing only excess heat clearing herbs will have only a partial effect and the fire will soon return. The addition of fang feng gives the ability to vent heat upwards and outwards. If fang feng is omitted, there will be no improvement.

Huo xiang is added for its aromatic ability to revive the spleen, remove turbid dampness, transform phlegm, and promote the flow of qi. Huo xiang makes for a wonderful addition to any formula when there is stagnation in the stomach with a weakened spleen.

Common spleen fire symptoms manifest as oral symptoms, including severe thirst and frequent hunger, mouth ulcers, bad breath, dry lips, a hot and dry tongue, and a rapid pulse.

YU NU JIAN

Yu Nu Jian 玉努煎 (Jade Woman Decoction) is a helpful standalone or additional formula to treat hot flashes. By draining heat from the stomach and nourishing kidney yin, it treats dual excess deficiency patterns by directing fire downward.

Herbs in the formula: shi gao, shu di huang, zhi mu, mai men dong, niu xi.

Vigorous stomach fire injures kidney yin. Shi gao clears fire from the heart and stomach, while shu di huang nourishes kidney water to restrain fire. As previously stated, hot flashes can be caused or agitated by fire in the stomach. Shi gao has an excellent ability to clear stomach fire.

Zhi mu helps clear heat due to stomach, lung, and kidney yin deficiency. Zhi mu is also moistening in nature and a better choice for clearing heat due to deficiency. Mai men dong helps moisten the stomach, generates fluids, and alleviates irritability. Niu xi conducts heat downwards.

Common stomach heat manifestations include toothache, bleeding gums, frontal headaches, a red tongue and a dry, yellow coating, a floating, slippery, and large pulse, irritability, fever, and thirst. The strength of the pulse will depend upon the amount of kidney yin deficiency.

LONG DAN XIE GAN TANG

Long Dan Xie Gan Tang 龙担泻肝汤 (Gentianae Longdancao Decoction to Drain the Liver) treats hot flashes due to excess fire in the liver and gallbladder or smoldering damp-heat in the lower jiao. Although they do not directly generate hot flashes, these excess patterns have the tendency to rise up and agitate the heart fire.

Herbs in the formula: long dan cao, huang qin, zhi zi, chai hu, mu tong, che qian zi, ze xie, sheng di huang, dang gui, gan cao.

Long dan cao is very cold and bitter in nature and is the primary herb for draining excess heat or fire from the liver and gallbladder and for eliminating damp-heat in the lower jiao. Much like many of the previously discussed cold herbs, long dan cao will cause spleen deficiency and is not a good choice for long-term use.

As previously described, huang qin and zhi zi are added to help drain fire from all three jiao. Mu tong, che qian zi, and ze xie are a powerful combination and aid in draining fire and damp-heat by promoting diuresis. Without these herbs in the formula, the heat would have nowhere to go and would cause further complications.

Sheng di huang and dang gui supplement yin and nourish blood. They are very effective at protecting against the harsh heat clearing herbs. Chai hu is a principal herb for dispersing heat due to constrained liver and gallbladder qi. Chai hu and huang qin is a classic combination for clearing shaoyang channel heat.

Constrained heat or fire in the liver and gallbladder channels blazes upwards, causing manifestations such as chest tightness, hypochondria pain, headache, dizziness, red and sore eyes, hearing loss, a bitter taste, irritability and short temper, and a wiry and rapid pulse. Damp-heat flows from the liver meridian into the lower jiao and causes leukorrhea, a shortened menstrual cycle, turbid urination, and swelling and itching of the genitalia.

QING SHU YI QI TANG

Qing Shu Yi Qi Tang 清暑益气汤 (Clear Summer-Heat and Augment the Qi Decoction) is a traditional chao re tidal heat effusion formula. This is the "Wang Shi" version from the *Warp and Woof on Warm-Febrile Diseases* by Wang Mengying, 1852. This type of tidal heat effusion is a damp-evil obstruction pattern where hot and humid weather of late-summer penetrates and enters the body, impairing the spleen and stomach qi and body fluids.

Even though this formula is able to treat tidal heat effusion, it is seldom used because summer-heat is rarely at the center of the hot-flash environment. It may be of use for women who are susceptible to pronounced or an increase in hot flashes during the summer months or when living in a hot and damp climate.

Qing Shu Yi Qi Tang actions are to clear summer-heat, augment qi, nourish yin, and generate fluids for treating summer-heat patterns.

Herbs in the formula: xi yang shen, shi hu, mai men dong, xi gua pi, he geng, zhu ye, zhi mu, huang lian, gan cao, geng mi.

Xi yang shen or American ginseng is an excellent herb that simultaneously clears heat and tonifies qi, yin, and body fluids. It is surprising that this herb is not used more often in hot-flash formulas. Shi hu and mai men dong support xi yang shen by augmenting qi, generating fluids, nourishing lung and stomach yin, and clearing heat.

Xi gua pi and he geng are for clearing heat and releasing summer-heat. Zhu ye and zhi mu are added for their heat clearing actions and ability to resolve irritability and thirst. A very small dose of huang lian is added to aid in quelling fire. Gan cao and geng mi too augment qi and nourish the stomach. They help prevent the cloying nature of yin nourishing herbs and protect from the cold nature of the heat clearing herbs.

Manifestations include fever, profuse sweating, irritability, thirst, scanty urine, desire to curl up, shortness of breath, apathy, and a weak and rapid pulse.

An original formula carrying the same name, Qing Shu Yi Qi Tang, known as the "Li" version, dates back to the *Pi Wei Lun* by Li Dong

Yuan, 1249. The main difference between the two is that the former addresses summer-heat patterns from a febrile-disease standpoint while the latter addresses qi deficiency patterns complicated by an attack of summer-heat.

Li's original version can be adopted to treat hot flashes due to qi deficiency generating smoldering yin fire within the mingmen.

Repletion and Stagnation Prescriptions
Treating Repletion and Stagnation Patterns

This section covers herbal formulas that treat repletion and stagnation patterns and includes qi stagnation, blood stasis, and phlegm and dampness accumulation, along with digestive and other related chronic conditions. These formulas treat repletion and stagnation patterns where it is necessary to regulate qi and allow free flow of qi, blood, and body fluids to resume.

Two formulas mentioned in the *Shang Han Lun* section are covered, along with several formulas dealing with repletion and stagnation in various parts of the zangfu system with a variety of causes.

Many stagnation issues happen over time, but some can happen more abruptly. Repletion and stagnation patterns primarily develop over a background of deficiency or as a result of a combination of environmental factors, emotional stressors, and lifestyle and dietary habits.

Heat and fire are not the center of repletion and stagnation patterns but are often a manifestation or result of the built up or blocked qi. In these cases, treating hot-flash patients can be confusing because oftentimes the practitioner can see the signs of deficiency and may think the heat effusion is a result of deficiency heat, when in reality, the heat is the result of the repletion or stagnation.

It is vital that the practitioner checks for repletion and stagnation issues during diagnosis. If there are repletion and stagnation issues, it is necessary to address them first or in conjunction with any other underlying issues. If not, the repletion and stagnation patterns will continue generating heat and consuming vital qi.

Cases of early menopausal transition issues are on the rise. It is important to understand that the ovarian reserve is a part of the jing (essence). Jing, qi, and blood are consumed at a much more rapid rate than normal. Some of the women in this category have started life with a lower-than-normal ovarian reserve, which places them in the jing deficiency or pre-heaven qi deficiency constitution. But in general, a life of repletion and stagnation due to lifestyle issues will consume jing at a much more rapid rate than normal. This is because repletion and stagnation obstruct qi and blood flow, yin and yang balance, and the entire zangfu system, leading to dysfunction. Dysfunction, along with heat or fire development from the repletion and stagnation, is the fuel to drive unnecessary consumption of the vital qi.

Repletion and stagnation patterns can also be the result of pre-heaven qi or genetic issues creating predisposition. This is seen in people who generally gravitate towards certain habitual problems. It is usually seen in digestive problems, breathing problems, emotional problems, or energy-level problems that begin during the early years of one's life. For example, it is necessary to question if constipation developed as a child, as a teenager, in college, or as an adult. This will present a complete story as to whether it's a result of a genetic predisposition, stress, hormone factors, or other related lifestyle habits. In any case, it is still necessary to promote and support the digestive process, but the cause of the underlying issue will steer the treatment.

The practitioner needs to be able to diagnose and distinguish between a deficiency constitution and one of repletion and stagnation that has consumed the jing. Repletion and stagnation patterns are often the main cause of perimenopausal or early menopausal transition issues such as irregular periods, heavy or consistent bleeding, bleeding between periods, mood and sleep issues, and hot flashes. When women seek out "hormone imbalance" and early menopausal transition treatments between their late thirties and mid-forties, I usually look for signs of repletion and stagnation before anything else. There is also a small percentage of women who will enter into early menopausal transition in their forties when ovarian reserve has declined at a much more rapid rate and earlier than normal.

Repletion and stagnation formulas can be strong at moving qi and blood, descending qi, and resolving damp and phlegm. It is necessary to take precautions when treating women who may be pregnant, women who have excessive bleeding, and women with vital qi deficiency.

- Da Cheng Qi Tang

- Xiao Chai Hu Tang

- Xiao Yao San

- Huo Xiang Zheng Qi San

- Xue Fu Zhu Yu Tang

- Er Chen Tang

- Wen Dan Tang.

DA CHENG QI TANG

Da Cheng Qi Tang 大承气汤 (Major Order Qi Decoction) is a powerful herbal formula for purging internal excess heat, specifically from the yangming stomach and large intestine fu organs. This is known as yangming fu syndrome and was described almost 2000 years ago in the *Shang Han Lun*.

Constitutional or genetic factors, lifestyle habits, or vital qi deficiency can cause stagnation development within the yangming fu organs, which blocks qi and generates internal excess heat. Da Cheng Qi Tang is a classic formula for treating constipation.

Herbs in the formula: da huang, mang xiao, zhi shi, hou po.

Repletion, stagnation, and heat within the yangming fu organs injures and consumes yin and body fluids, dries out the stool, and results in severe or chronic constipation and frequent gas. Yangming fu syndrome will generate tidal fever that is more pronounced around 3–5pm, along with sweating of the hands and feet.

Internal excess heat can easily aggravate the hot-flash environment, pushing relatively mild hot flashes into a moderate to severe category. Internal heat repletion can ascend and harass the heart fire, causing hot flashes and other menopausal-transition symptoms such as anxiety, palpitations, and insomnia. Many hot-flash scenarios subside once the internal excess heat is purged. This is a habitual pattern, and in some situations continual purging of this accumulated heat is necessary. Constitutional deficiencies and lifestyle issues need to be addressed in order to break the cycle.

Patients with yangming excess can have constipation and dry stools accompanied by the four types of abdominal disharmony: distension, fullness, dryness, and hardness. Yangming excess presents with a prickled tongue with a thick coating and a deep, slippery, and forceful pulse.

Da huang is a very bitter and cold herb that's able to drain heat and stagnation from the yangming fu organs. Mang xiao is added as an adjuvant purgative and helps moisten dryness within the digestive tract. These herbs make a perfect pair for constipation. Zhi shi and hou po are two strong-acting herbs that are added to the formula and are especially helpful in resolving qi stagnation within the abdomen and digestive tract.

It is important not to use Da Cheng Qi Tang during pregnancy because of its purging nature or in patients with weak constitutions where it will further injure vital qi. Its lesser formula Xiao Cheng Qi Tang eliminates mang xiao from the formula and is suitable for mild excess heat patterns or in patients with weaker constitutions.

XIAO CHAI HU TANG

Xiao Chai Hu Tang 小柴胡汤 (Minor Bupleurum Decoction) is a classic formula from the *Shang Han Lun* that mediates or harmonizes shaoyang or half interior half exterior disease. The shaoyang is halfway between the exterior (yang) and interior (yin). Many diseases, whether coming from the exterior or interior, can lodge or stick within the shaoyang, creating difficult and stubborn qi stagnation issues.

Shaoyang is known for its chronicity and is often due to an excess/deficiency situation.

Some hot-flash patients will present with various stubborn or chronic symptoms that have eluded effective relief from previous treatments.

Shaoyang is affiliated with the gallbladder fu organ which is interior-exterior related to the liver zang organ. Liver and gallbladder qi stagnation issues are often the root problem behind the shaoyang syndrome, leading to the generation of heat.

The heart, liver, and stomach are all prone to fire. If the liver and gallbladder become stagnant and overheated, they will generate issues along the liver and gallbladder channels that affect the head and harass the stomach and heart zangfu organs. This is how shaoyang issues generate and agitate the hot-flash environment. It is threefold: yin and yang are thrown out of balance and affect the brain and HPO axis; heat repletion agitates the heart fire; the kidney and spleen are further weakened by the overaction of the liver and gallbladder.

Herbs in the formula: chai hu, huang qin, ban xia, sheng jiang, ren shen, zhi gan cao, da zao.

Xiao Chai Hu Tang is a well-designed formula to address the complicated excess deficiency, exterior-interior shaoyang disorders. Chai hu is the main herb to resolve this issue and is able to vent the exterior, resolving liver qi stagnation. Huang qin is added for its ability to purge the interior and clear gallbladder heat. Together, these two herbs harmonize the shaoyang. Ban xia harmonizes and directs stomach excess downwards. This is beneficial in redirecting qi away from the heart. Ren shen strongly supports the vital qi, while the rest of the herbs help balance and harmonize the actions of the main herbs.

The beautiful nature of Chinese medicine is its amazing effectiveness in treating these types of situations by reducing excess, regulating qi, and clearing heat while simultaneously nourishing deficiency.

Classic shaoyang symptoms include alternating fever and chills, fullness in the chest and hypochondrium with difficulty in taking deep breaths, interior heat rising, a bitter taste in the mouth, a dry throat, dizziness, heartburn, frequent nausea, poor appetite, and a wiry pulse. Pay attention to these symptoms and patients with frequent dysregulation of body temperature.

XIAO YAO SAN

Xiao Yao San 逍遥散 (Rambling Powder) is one of the world's most popular Chinese herbal formulas. This is because it can easily correct liver and spleen disharmony. This pattern is commonly seen in today's society as a result of the stressors of everyday emotional and dietary activity. Xiao Yao San is commonly prescribed for emotional instability and premenstrual syndrome, and is often used prophylactically.

Once the liver and spleen fall out of balance, the liver is apt to excess and stagnation while the spleen is prone to weakness. When the liver qi becomes stagnant, it overreacts on the spleen, causing a decline in its ability to produce qi and blood. This situation puts further stress on the kidney-liver-spleen triad, already prone to deficiency, and eventually results in blood deficiency. A blood deficient (yin) environment allows an excess qi (yang) environment to develop naturally within the liver, giving rise to the development of liver fire. The ascending nature of liver fire can easily harass the heart fire, thus generating or agitating the hot-flash environment.

Xiao Yao San relieves stagnation of liver qi and strengthens the spleen to nourish blood. Liver qi stagnation with concurrent blood deficiency is a common pattern seen in today's society and can naturally ensue over time due to decades of a menstrual cycle. It is vital for women to have an abundant and healthy supply of blood for a smooth menopausal transition.

Herbs in the formula: chai hu, bo he, dang gui, bai shao, bai zhu, fu ling, zhi gan cao, wei jiang.

Chai hu dredges the flow of liver qi to relieve stagnation. Bo he is mint and is cooling in nature and added to help soothe the flow of liver qi and disperse heat. Mint tea can be consumed to relieve mild cases of qi stagnation. Dang gui and bai shao nourish blood and soften liver qi. This is important because liver qi stagnation often develops because of liver blood deficiency. Bai zhu, fu ling, zhi gan cao, and wei jiang tonify the spleen and stomach to generate qi and blood and prevent the liver from overacting on the spleen.

Common manifestations include pain along the ribs and hypochondrium, distended breasts, premenstrual tension, irregular menstruation, shaoyang disease (alternating fever and chills and a bitter taste), headaches, vertigo, a dry mouth and throat, fatigue, reduced appetite, a pale red tongue, and a wiry pulse.

Jia Wei Xiao Yao San is a common modified formula and is perhaps prescribed more often than the traditional formula. It has the addition of mu dan pi and zhi zi to help clear the constrained heat from liver qi stagnation.

This is a brilliant formula that has the ability to help relieve many hot-flash and menopausal-transition patterns. Practitioners need to understand that this formula, along with these two herbs in particular, moves qi and blood and clears heat. On the plus side, the formula relieves the symptoms, but on the downside, its use over time can have a detrimental effect of weakening qi and yin. The formula Yi Guan Jian is better suited to liver and kidney yin deficiency with concurrent liver qi stagnation.

Chai Hu Shu Gan San is a stronger formula for regulating and moving liver qi. It is necessary to use Chai Hu Shu Gan San over Xiao Yao San for robust liver qi stagnation patterns without concurrent spleen qi deficiency (there have been several hot-flash cases in my clinic where it was necessary to do this). These patients are often calm and focused yet demanding and quite easily agitated.

Qi stagnation with yin deficiency case study: A 53-year-old female patient presented with moderate nighttime hot flashes and night sweating for one year. Accompanying symptoms included skin itchiness, especially on the legs, acid reflux, high stress levels, minor fatigue, and a history of allergies. The patient otherwise led a clean and healthy lifestyle. Her pulse was rapid and thin. Her tongue was puffy and pale with a red tip.

I originally diagnosed her with yin and blood deficiency with qi stagnation. The patient was unable to receive acupuncture treatments and wanted to utilize Chinese herbal medicine. The patient was prescribed Tu Fu Ling Sheng Di Huang. After one week, the patient's skin conditions subsided; however, the hot flashes and stress levels remained high. The patient was prescribed Jia Wei Xiao Yao San and Zuo Gui Wan. The hot flashes and night sweats resolved and the patient's stress levels returned to normal after two weeks.

Yin and blood deficiency with qi stagnation is a classic hot-flash environment pattern and many patients respond well to these two formulas when they are used together. Zuo Gui Wan addresses the underlying root deficiency of yin and blood deficiency, while Jia Wei Xiao Yao San addresses stress and lifestyle-induced symptoms seen in menopausal-transition patients.

HUO XIANG ZHENG QI SAN

Huo Xiang Zheng Qi San 霍香正气散 (Agastache Powder to Rectify the Qi) releases the exterior, transforms dampness, regulates qi, and harmonizes the middle jiao. This formula does not specifically address hot flashes, as it does not clear heat, but it does treat the root of many hot-flash environments, which is dampness and stagnation in the middle jiao. This type of pattern disrupts the spleen's ability to produce fresh qi and blood and blocks the descending stomach qi, resulting in rebellious and ascending qi.

Traditionally, Huo Xiang Zheng Qi San is used for treating sudden digestive diseases such as abdominal pain, vomiting, and diarrhea, due to the stomach flu, unsanitary food or poor water conditions, parasites, or hot and damp weather. Whichever the cause, the stomach and spleen are affected and lose their ability to transform and transport food and water. The spleen becomes weak and loses its ability to move body fluids, resulting in dampness accumulation, while the stomach qi becomes knotted and is unable to descend.

The result is chronic damp stagnation which, over time, affects the yin and yang balance, qi and blood circulation, and communication within the rest of the zangfu organs. Most often, the immediate symptoms decline, while chronic low-grade digestive and qi stagnation symptoms remain and develop. This is why it is necessary to diagnose and treat the digestive tract. Chronic conditions ensue if the transportation and transformation functions of the spleen and stomach are left unresolved.

Herbs in the formula: huo xiang, hou po, chen pi, zi su ye, bai zhi, ban xia, da fu pi, bai zhu, fu ling, jie geng, zhi gan cao, sheng jiang, da zao.

The chief herbs huo xiang, hou po, chen pi, and fu ling rectify knotted stomach qi and resolve dampness in the middle jiao with their strong aromatic nature and qi moving actions. It is vital to rectify the knotted stomach qi. If not, stagnant stomach qi has the tendency to ascend and exuberant yang qi or fire can rise and affect the heart.

The rest of the formula is composed of two smaller formulas, Ping Wei San and Er Chen Tang, which focus on drying dampness, improving spleen transporting function, promoting movement of qi, and harmonizing the stomach.

Huo Xiang Zheng Qi San works very well and is usually only needed for a short time. Menopausal-transition symptoms will respond and lessen once chronic qi stagnation and dampness accumulation in the middle jiao is resolved.

XUE FU ZHU YU TANG

Xue Fu Zhu Yu Tang 血俯逐淤汤 (Drive Out Stasis in the Mansion of Blood Decoction) is the main formula designed for treating blood stasis and qi stagnation patterns. Its actions are to invigorate blood, transform stasis, spread liver qi, and unblock the channels. Once the qi circulates, the blood will circulate. Qi is the commander of blood and blood is the mother of qi.

Xue Fu Zhu Yu Tang both moves qi and invigorates blood. It is mainly used for relieving pain, but it can also treat many menopausal-transition symptoms including palpitations, insomnia, irritability, depression, tidal fever, and irregular periods, resulting from blood stasis and qi stagnation blocking and preventing nourishment from reaching the heart. Blood stasis and qi stagnation are often chronic in nature and take a long time to develop.

Using blood invigorating formulas can be intimidating for some practitioners and can lead to worries about causing harm to patients. The truth is, however, that blood invigorating formulas are well designed and very safe to use, even when they are needed for long-term care. One detail to remember is that the root cause of many blood stasis patterns is qi and blood deficiency. It will be necessary to look for the appropriate signs and treat accordingly. Xue Fu Zhu Yu Tang and many of its modifications can treat the root cause of many long-standing and complicated cases.

Herbs in the formula: tao ren, hong hua, chuan xiong, chi shao, dang gui, sheng di huang, chai hu, zhi ke, jie geng, niu xi, gan cao.

Tao ren and hong hua are two primary herbs that invigorate blood and dispel stasis. These herbs are sometimes enough to treat uncomplicated blood stasis patterns. They are often added to the blood tonic Si Wu

Tang to create Tao Hong Si Wu Tang, a simple and elegant formula that addresses blood deficiency with concurrent blood stasis.

Chuan xiong, chi shao, dang gui, and sheng di huang not only invigorate blood, they also nourish blood and clear heat. Chai hu, zhi ke, jie geng, and niu xi synergistically work together to rectify and balance yin and yang and facilitate the movement of qi.

Xue Fu Zhu Yu Tang has many modifications that address blood stasis and qi stagnation in different areas of the body. For example, Tong Qiao Huo Xue Tang treats the head, face, and upper parts of the body. Ge Xia Zhu Yu Tang treats diaphragm and upper abdominal issues. Shao Fu Zhu Yu Tang treats lower abdominal and uterine issues. Shen Tong Zhu Yu Tang treats aches and pain in the extremities.

ER CHEN TANG

Er Chen Tang 二陈汤 (Two Cured Decoction) is a universal formula to treat dampness and phlegm. It is often used as a standalone formula or in conjunction with other formulas. Damp-phlegm accumulates when qi is unable to propel and circulate body fluids or when there is deficiency in the lung-spleen-kidney axis, the primary zangfu organs in charge of water metabolism. When the spleen fails to transport body fluids, they accumulate to form damp-phlegm. Damp-phlegm in turn interferes with the spleen's ability to properly function, creating a vicious cycle.

Qi deficiency is usually the root cause, while damp-phlegm accumulation is the manifestation. That is why the preferred treatment for damp-phlegm is to strengthen the spleen by regulating qi.

Damp-phlegm is quite common but can complicate the hot-flash environment. It manifests in many forms such as focal distension and stifling sensation in the chest and diaphragm, palpitations, dizziness, chronic sinus issues and allergies, post-nasal drip, coughing with phlegm, nausea, a slippery pulse, and a swollen tongue with a white, thick, and greasy coating. It is quite easy, though, to improve the situation by strengthening the spleen and rectifying qi.

Herbs in the formula: ban xia, ju hong, fu ling, zhi gan cao, sheng jiang, wu mei.

Ban xia dries dampness, expels phlegm, and directs rebellious stomach qi downwards. It treats vomiting, nausea, and acid reflux due to knotted stomach qi, as well as asthma and chronic lung conditions due to lung qi unable to descend. Ju hong revives the spleen and facilitates qi flow in the middle jiao. Fu ling is perhaps the most versatile herb for treating dampness by inducing diuresis and strengthening the spleen. Fu ling also has the function of calming the spirit. It is worth mentioning the holy herb for treating stomach disorders, sheng jiang. It soothes and rectifies the stomach qi and warms and strengthens the middle jiao. Altogether, Er Chen Tang is a remarkable formula for treating sluggish, weak, and problematic hot-flash environments.

WEN DAN TANG

Wen Dan Tang 温胆汤 (Warm the Gallbladder Decoction) is a modification of Er Chen Tang, adding the two herbs zhu ru and zhi shi. This changes the focus to treating damp-phlegm accumulation with heat repletion mainly in the gallbladder and stomach. Wen Dan Tang regulates qi, transforms phlegm, clears the gallbladder, and harmonizes the stomach.

Increased and prolonged qi stagnation in the middle jiao and spleen qi deficiency often affect these two fu organs, creating a chronic phlegm-heat pattern. Phlegm-heat is a relatively common hot-flash environment pattern where the excess heat and qi stagnation within these two organs rises and disturbs the heart and chest, causing hot flashes, irritability, insomnia, palpitations, anxiety, and increased heat manifestations. A patient's tongue may be red if heat is significant or pale if there is considerable qi deficiency. The tongue coating will be dry, coarse, and yellow, and the pulse will be more rapid.

Zhu ru is the main herb for clearing heat and phlegm in the gallbladder and stomach. It reverses the rebellious flow of stomach qi and relieves restlessness. The addition of zhi shi enhances the flow of qi to dissolve phlegm.

Qi and Blood Deficiency Prescriptions

Qi and blood deficiency is one of the leading problems that creates a hot-flash environment and is possibly even more prevalent than yin deficiency. Qi and blood deficiency can easily become a problem, but thankfully, this is easily resolvable.

Qi Deficiency Hot Flashes

Qi deficiency tidal heat effusion develops when qi is weak and yang qi is unable to ascend and sinks into yin. This is the result of dietary and lifestyle habits damaging the lung and spleen taiyin. When taiyin are weak, they can no longer support the rising of qi, which allows yang qi to sink into yin.

In this qi deficient state, wei qi and yang qi are weak and cannot circulate and therefore cannot warm and protect the body. This leaves the body susceptible to cold and pathogenic invasion. When yang qi sinks into yin within the lower jiao, it warms the mingmen fire and generates heat. This is a source of low-grade tidal heat effusion. This type of tidal heat effusion is commonly seen during the morning when yang qi is beginning its ascent.

This pattern causes generalized heat effusion, heart vexation, spontaneous sweating, aversion to cold, fatigue, and a surging forceless pulse.

Blood and Yin Deficiency Hot Flashes

Blood deficiency tidal heat effusion develops when yin qi is deficient and unable to fill the vessels and cool the tissues. This is a common result of blood loss from the menstrual cycle, trauma, severe illness, or spleen deficiency being unable to generate new blood. When yin and blood are deficient, they are unable to cool the body and constrain yang qi. Yang qi and wei qi are left unabated and are able to roam and circulate freely. By doing so, their natural tendency to warm the body increases, causing heat effusion, especially in the evening when yin and blood are more susceptible to deficiency.

The opposite to qi deficiency, this pattern causes generalized heat effusion, a red complexion, thirst, heart vexation, night sweating, agitation, insomnia, and a surging forceless pulse.

Tonifying herbs and prescriptions are used for treating the hot-flash environment in the following ways: nourish and support a healthy zangfu organ environment to generate vital qi; clear excess and deficiency heat; maintain yin and yang balance; return balance to water and fire.

There are two main tonification categories: qi and blood; yin and yang. Tonification is often centralized on the lung, spleen, and kidney as the main organs of pre-heaven and post-heaven qi. Qi tonics focus on the spleen and lung. Blood tonics focus on the heart and liver. Yin tonics focus on the liver and kidney. Yang tonics focus on the kidney. There is a myriad of tonic formulas with similar functions and indications.

- Bu Zhong Yi Qi Tang

- Si Wu Tang

- Dang Gui Bu Xue Tang.

BU ZHONG YI QI TANG
Bu Zhong Yi Qi Tang 补中益气汤 (Tonify the Middle and Augment the Qi Decoction) is the principal formula from the *Pi Wei Lun*. Its central focus is tonifying the middle jiao and raising sunken yang qi, and it treats general spleen and stomach qi deficiency.

Spleen and stomach qi deficiency is often the central issue of the hot-flash environment. It is easy in today's demanding and draining society for them to become weakened, especially in women, since they need to continually resupply qi and blood after every menstrual cycle. The organs are unable to generate qi and blood when they are weak. They are left unable to redeem the quantities of qi and blood, leaving a general emptiness. Qi deficiency gives rise to mild heat symptoms and spontaneous sweating.

Diagnosing qi and blood deficiency in hot-flash patients by simply looking at the complexion is quite easy: it should generally be pale. The pulse may be slow or fast depending on the overall situation of the yang qi and relative stagnation or heat signs generated by the deficiency; however, the overall strength will be forceless and weak. The key to treating hot flashes is deciding when to nourish and when to clear. Though not commonly thought of when treating hot flashes, Bu Zhong Yi Qi Tang can be very useful because it builds healthy qi and blood supplies, raises yang, and fills up the vessels and zangfu organs, thus abating heat.

Herbs in the formula: huang qi, ren shen, bai zhu, zhi gan cao, dang gui, chen pi, sheng ma, chai hu.

Huang qi is a powerful qi tonic and strengthens the vital qi, which helps strengthen the wei qi and raises yang qi to abate hot flashes. Ren shen, bai zhu, and zhi gan cao are a reliable combination to strengthen the spleen qi, vital qi, and the middle jiao. They compose the basic qi tonic formula Si Jun Zi Tang and are utilized to treat the underlying deficiency. Dang gui is a warming blood tonic that helps strengthen qi.

Sheng ma and chai hu help huang qi with their ascending ability to lift sunken yang qi. If they are not used, the yang qi will stay within the yin aspects and have difficulty rising.

A deficiency of qi cannot ascend to support lucid yang. Yang sinks into the yin and is unable to circulate, protect, and warm the superficial levels. Tidal heat is thus generated within the yin. This type of low-grade fever is intermittent with an on-again, off-again nature and is worse on exertion. It is accompanied by spontaneous sweating and an aversion to cold. A thirst for warm beverages and tongue and pulse signs will distinguish this pattern from yin deficiency. I've treated many hot-flash cases due to qi deficiency with Bu Zhong Yi Qi Tang. I was doubtful at first, but when the pattern is correct, the herbs work.

It is useful to know and understand qi tonic formulas and their properties when treating the hot-flash environment. Some commonly used qi deficiency prescriptions include Si Jun Zi Tang and its affiliations, Shen Ling Bai Zhu San, Sheng Mai San, and Li Zhong Wan. These formulas tend to be warming and drying in nature with little or no yin nourishing properties. If they are not properly modified or utilized with another formula, it is unwise to administer them to patients with yin deficiency or heat patterns.

SI WU TANG

Si Wu Tang 四物汤 (Four Herb Decoction) is the main herbal formula that tonifies blood. Nourishing blood in menopausal women and in women in general is essential. Building blood regulates the liver, supports the heart, and strengthens the chong and ren vessels.

Irregular periods during the early stages of menopausal transition are normal. It is essential to nourish blood to strengthen the liver, along with the chong and ren vessels, to support the uterus and help maintain a smooth menstrual cycle all the way to the FMP. Spirit disturbances including anxiety and insomnia commonly increase through menopausal transition. It is important to nourish heart blood to support and calm the shen.

Herbs in the formula: shu di huang, bai shao, dang gui, chuan xiong.

Shu di huang is a powerful herb that tonifies yin and blood by strengthening its foundation from the liver and kidney. Blood and yin are of the same source. It nourishes the yin of blood. Bai shao is cool in nature and a strong addition to nourish the yin of blood. Dang gui is slightly warm and has the function of circulating blood. It is used to both tonify and invigorate blood. It nourishes the yang of blood. The final ingredient, chuan xiong, invigorates blood and promotes the movement of qi. It is essential to release areas of qi constraint, especially in the liver. Qi is susceptible to stagnation when the blood is deficient. Qi cannot move without blood and they rely on each other. Dang gui and chuan xiong help offset the rich and cloying nature and stagnating properties of shu di huang and bai shao.

Si Wu Tang is a safe standalone formula that can be used long term with menopausal-transition patients to treat many symptoms, including hot flashes. Its four ingredients can be found in numerous formulas, including yin tonics for treating the hot-flash environment.

It's worth noting that blood and yin tonics need to be used with caution in patients with significant qi deficiency because of their stagnating nature, which can harm the spleen and stomach. This is why it is quite common to combine qi and blood tonic formulas. A prime example is combining the qi tonic Si Jun Zi Tang and the blood tonic Si Wu Tang to make Ba Zhen Tang.

DANG GUI BU XUE TANG

Dang Gui Bu Xue Tang 当归补血汤 (Tangkuei Decoction to Tonify the Blood) is the preferred and elegant qi and blood tonification formula. This is a remarkable formula to support qi and blood deficiency due to overexertion and overtaxation.

The potential value of this formula from a hot-flash perspective arises because when both qi and blood become deficient, yang qi can erratically sink into yin or float towards the surface. Yang qi is warm in nature. When the yang qi sinks into yin it resides, warms, and then bursts to the surface. Conversely, when the yang qi is floating, it will bring extra warmth to the surface in the form of tidal heat effusion or hot flashes.

Herbs in the formula: huang qi, dang gui.

This formula uses only two ingredients: huang qi to tonify qi and dang gui to tonify blood. Huang qi reinforces the lung and spleen to generate qi to reinforce the source of blood. Dang gui tonifies and invigorates blood for better generation of new blood. The special attention in this formula is the 5:1 huang qi to dang gui ratio of herbs to powerfully nourish the source qi to generate new blood. At first glance, it would appear that the use of huang qi would accentuate ascending yang qi and heat sensations; however, it abates heat sensations by lifting sinking yang qi from smoldering within yin and strengthens yang to generate yin or blood, thus balancing ascending yang qi and heat.

The texts state that Dang Gui Bu Xue Tang is contraindicated in patients with yin deficiency heat. Therefore, this formula must only be used in treating patients with qi and blood deficiency. However, yin and blood are of the same source and one inevitably affects the other. It is safer to say that what the texts imply is that the qi and blood are deficient, yet the source yin of the kidney is still intact.

When the deficient source qi leads to nutritive qi and blood deficiency, the weakened yin is unable to hold the yang, allowing for floating yang qi. Along with hot flashes, accompanying menopausal-transition symptoms include a red complexion and irritability.

The key to blood deficiency diagnosis is a pale tongue. The clue to yang qi rising due to deficiency is the surging and floating but forceless pulse.

Yin Deficiency Prescriptions

Yin deficiency empty heat patterns and hot flashes are often thought of as being synonymous in modern Chinese medicine. This is not entirely correct. A more accurate understanding is that empty heat patterns exacerbate the hot-flash environment. Yin nourishing and empty heat clearing formulas can be used to treat the imbalance within the hot-flash environment to quell the hot flash.

Relative and True Yin Nourishing Prescriptions

There are two types of yin deficiency formulas: one for relative yin deficiency and one for true or absolute yin deficiency. As previously discussed, relative yin deficiency materializes in the zangfu organs and has particular and individual effects on the liver, heart, spleen, lung, and kidney. Yin deficiency has the natural tendency to generate heat. As the yin (water) declines, the yang (fire) increases. This yin deficient heat can be mild or particularly intense in nature and, over time, slowly dries out the organs and tissues. Over time, relative yin deficiency will eventually affect and injure the true yin of the kidney.

True yin deficiency, on the other hand, is the decline of the original yin and essence of the kidney. This original or true yin is the foundation and source of yin for the rest of the body. True yin deficiency may be congenital or the result of damage by severe illness or natural decline that occurs with age. True yin deficiency may have none or very minor deficiency heat signs or particularly intense and deep heat symptoms.

Relative yin deficiency and its heat symptoms often respond better to treatments because damage is not as severe. True yin deficiency, on the other hand, will take a longer approach to repair the damaged yin.

Yin Nourishing Versus Deficiency Heat Clearing Prescriptions

Yin deficiency formulas can be further broken down into two categories: those that nourish yin and those that clear deficiency heat. Most yin deficiency prescriptions fall somewhere along a spectrum between purely nourishing yin and purely clearing heat. This is apparent in the herbs that comprise the formulas.

- Zhi Bai Di Huang Wan

- Zuo Gui Wan

- Da Bu Yin Wan

- Er Zhi Wan

- Yi Guan Jian

- Er Xian Tang

- Qing Hao Bie Jia Tang

- Qing Gu San.

ZHI BAI DI HUANG WAN

Zhi Bai Di Huang Wan 知柏地黃丸 (Anemarrhena Phellodendron and Rehmannia Pill) nourishes liver and kidney yin and clears empty heat or deficiency fire, consumptive heat, and bone heat due to severe illness or yin deficiency. Adding zhi mu and huang bai makes it a modified variation on the classic yin deficiency formula Liu Wei Di Huang Wan. Zhi Bai Di Huang Wan is considered a classic foundational formula for treating menopausal transition.

Herbs in the formula: shu di huang, shan zhu yu, shan yao, ze xie, mu dan pi, fu ling, zhi mu, huang bai.

The first step in quelling fire is building up the yin reserves. Fire cannot burn brightly if water is abundant. The first three herbs in the formula are tonic herbs that nourish kidney and liver yin and the spleen qi.

The second step in quelling fire is draining residual fire. The second group of herbs functions to clear heat due to deficiency by draining liver and kidney fire.

The final two herbs zhi mu and huang bai strengthen the formula's clearing of deficiency fire. Zhi mu and huang bai are often paired and can be added to any formula, including qi and blood tonics, to achieve this desired effect.

Yin deficiency over time generates classic internal deficiency heat signs such as a red tongue with little moisture and no coating, a thin and rapid pulse, irritability, a flushed face, a chronic sore throat, and heat on the soles, palms, and center of the chest.

It is worth noting that sometimes menopausal-transition patients will present in the clinic with concurrent kidney yin deficiency and hyperactive liver fire. This concurrent pattern responds well to combining Zhi Bai Di Huang Wan with Long Dan Xie Gan Tang.

ZUO GUI WAN
Zuo Gui Wan 左归丸 (Restore the Left (Kidney) Pill) functions to nourish and supplement kidney essence in cases of true or absolute yin deficiency. This is a different approach to treating the hot-flash environment than that of Zhi Bai Di Huang Wan. Zuo Gui Wan focuses on treating the deeper yin and yang properties of the kidney essence. Even though there are no fire draining or empty heat clearing herbs in the formula, once the essence is supported, Zuo Gui Wan indirectly abates heat manifestations that contribute to the hot-flash environment.

Herbs in the formula: shu di huang, gou qi zi, shan zhu yu, gui ban, lu jiao jiao, tu si zi, niu xi, shan yao.

Similar to Zhi Bai Di Huang Wan, Zuo Gui Wan tonifies the liver, kidney, and spleen with shu di huang, shan zhu yu, and shan yao, but adds gou qi zi, tu si zi, and niu xi to enhance the liver and kidney yin nourishing actions.

The real genius of this formula comes from the addition of gui ban and lu jiao jiao. These two herbs greatly nourish the yin and yang aspects of the kidney essence. Much like the theory from the Fire Spirit School, the yang strengthening function of lu jiao jiao helps guide any fire back to the source. This is especially useful in treating hot flashes. My experience indicates that using Zuo Gui Wan is effective in more hot-flash cases than using Zhi Bai Di Huang Wan.

DA BU YIN WAN

Da Bu Yin Wan 大补阴丸 (Great Tonify the Yin Pill) enriches the liver and kidney yin (water) and sedates deficiency fire. This formula is similar in structure to Zhi Bai Di Huang Wan and has a stronger effect clinically on treating deficiency fire manifestations.

Herbs in the formula: shu di huang, gui ban, huang bai, zhi mu.

This formula combines shu di huang and gui ban to greatly nourish yin and anchor yang. Huang bai sedates and zhi mu clears deficiency fire.

Da Bu Yin Wan can be used as a standalone formula or can be added to or used with other formulas. The theory is to "cultivate the root" by nourishing and enriching kidney yin and "clear the source" by clearing heat from the kidney. Both effects are necessary for successful treatment.

Upward rising of fire due to liver and kidney deficiency manifests with symptoms such as tidal fever, night sweats, and, in severe cases, bone heat. The rising fire can disturb the heart spirit, causing hot flashes, irritability, anxiety, and insomnia.

ER ZHI WAN

Er Zhi Wan 二侄丸 (Two Ultimate Pill) is a two-herb formula that treats kidney and liver yin deficiency. It is a common additive to other formulas for tonifying liver and kidney yin.

Herbs in the formula: nu zhen zi, han lian cao.

There are two important and beautiful aspects to this formula. First, neither herb is heavy nor cloying in nature. They are able to nourish both the kidney and liver yin without stagnating qi or having a negative impact on spleen qi. This makes it safe for long-term use. Second, both herbs are cool in nature and have the natural ability to cool residual deficiency heat in the patient.

This is an important formula during menopausal transition, as it is able to treat chronic uterine bleeding, general dryness in the respiratory tract and urogenital region, dizziness, blurred vision, and insomnia.

YI GUAN JIAN

Yi Guan Jian 一贯煎 (Linking Decoction) functions to enrich yin and spread the liver qi for liver and kidney yin deficiency with concurrent liver qi stagnation. Both Yi Guan Jian and Xiao Yao San address liver qi stagnation. The difference between the two formulas is the former treats liver qi stagnation with an underlying liver and kidney yin deficiency, whereas the latter treats liver qi stagnation with an underlying blood and spleen deficiency. Therefore, if there are signs of qi and blood deficiency, it is better to use Xiao Yao San.

Herbs in the formula: sheng di huang, gou qi zi, sha shen, mai men dong, dang gui, chuan lian zi.

The herbs in Yi Guan Jian are focused on treating the liver qi, blood, and yin. Sheng di huang is used in place of shu di huang for its stronger ability to clear heat and cool blood. This is an important formula modification when treating hot flashes. Gou qi zi and dang gui further help to nourish liver blood.

The unique aspect of this formula is the use of sha shen and mai men dong, which address the nourishing of yin and body fluids in the stomach and lung. This combination is another important formula modification. Lung and stomach yin deficiency is almost always overlooked when treating hot flashes. The final herb, chuan lian zi, helps disperse liver qi stagnation and clears heat.

ER XIAN TANG

Er Xian Tang 二仙汤 (Two Immortal Decoction) tonifies kidney yin and yang deficiency and drains deficiency fire. This formula has been identified by some sources as the hot-flash formula. Comprised of three yang nourishing herbs, two heat draining herbs, and one blood nourishing herb, it addresses yin and yang deficiency and drains fire commonly present in the hot-flash environment.

Herbs in the formula: xian mao, yin yang huo, ba ji tian, huang bai, zhi mu, dang gui.

Xian mao and ba ji tian tonify kidney yang, while yin yang huo tonifies both kidney yin and yang and anchors ascending yang. Huang bai and zhi mu support by clearing deficiency fire, especially from the kidney.

Dang gui is uniquely added to nourish the blood (yin) to balance the yang properties within the formula. Its warm nature also balances the cold nature of the fire draining properties within the formula. Finally, dang gui supports the chong and ren vessels.

By simultaneously nourishing both yin and yang and draining fire, Er Xian Tang addresses not only yang deficiency symptoms like fatigue, depression, and urinary frequency, but also yin deficiency and deficiency fire harassing the heart fire symptoms like hot flashes, irritability, anxiety, and insomnia.

QING HAO BIE JIA TANG

Qing Hao Bie Jia Tang 青蒿鳖甲汤 (Artemisia Annua and Soft-Shelled Turtle Shell Decoction) nourishes yin and clears heat due to the consumption of yin fluids by the late stage of febrile disease or long-standing internal heat.

Patients in this category are often recovering from or have been through a severe illness such as cancer. They are often noticeably fatigued and suffer from chronic or long-standing heat manifestations. Patients in this category are diagnosed with hot flashes not attributed to menopausal transition.

Herbs in the formula: bie jia, qing hao, sheng di huang, zhi mu, mu dan pi.

Bie jia and qing hao are a very effective combination to clear hidden heat and vent heat from the body. Bie jia enters the nutritive (ying) and blood (xue) levels to clear hidden fire. Qing hao guides this fire out. Sheng di huang, zhi mu, and mu dan pi nourish yin, cool blood, and disperse and clear deficiency heat.

Yin and body fluids are easily damaged by heat pathogens. Yin deficiency gives rise to ascending yang and heat manifestations. Common presentations include night fever and morning coolness, no sweating due to yin and body fluids depletion, emaciation or weight loss, a red tongue with little coating, and a fine and rapid pulse.

QING GU SAN

Qing Gu San 请骨散 (Cool the Bones Powder) clears heat from deficiency and alleviates tidal fever. It is classically indicated in steaming bone disorder, a deep interior heat where patients describe the heat as coming from their bones. This is a yin deficiency heat due to consumptive or febrile disease.

Herbs in the formula: yin chai hu, zhi mu, hu huang lian, di gu pi, qing hao, qin jiao, zhi bie jia, gan cao.

Qing Gu San primarily utilizes deficiency heat clearing herbs and is less focused on nourishing yin to abate heat.

Yin chai hu is the primary herb to clear deficiency heat from the deepest regions of the body. Zhi mu is added to nourish yin and quell deficiency fire. Hu huang lian clears heat from the blood level. Di gu pi clears heat from the lung, liver, and kidney. Qing hao and qin jiao help clear and disperse heat from the deeper regions. Zhi bie jia nourishes yin and guides the formula's heat clearing properties to the deeper regions of the body. Gan cao harmonizes and protects the stomach.

Qing Gu San and Qing Hao Bie Jia Tang are similar in function. Both treat nighttime hot flashes due to yin deficient heat. Qing Hao Bie Jia Tang nourishes yin, disperses deficiency heat, and is suitable for heat due to late-stage febrile disease. Qing Gu San nourishes yin and blood, clears deficiency fire, and is the better formula for relieving bone heat and nighttime fever.

Both patterns are similar in nature and have similar manifestations. Qing Gu San presents with more of the traditional yin deficiency fire menopausal-transition symptoms including afternoon tidal fever, chronic fever, night sweats, irritability, insomnia, emaciation, lethargy, red lips, malar flush, thirst, a dry throat, a red tongue with little coating, and a thin and rapid pulse.

Yang Deficiency Prescriptions

In some cases, it is necessary to stoke the kidney yang in the hot-flash environment to stimulate yin generation and to ignite the spleen to generate qi and blood. In other cases, it is necessary to fortify and lead true yang back to the mingmen to control ministerial fire.

- Jin Gui Shen Qi Wan

- You Gui Wan.

JIN GUI SHEN QI WAN

Jin Gui Shen Qi Wan 金贵肾气丸 (Kidney Qi Pill from the Golden Cabinet) warms and tonifies the kidney yang. It is a slight variation of Ba Wei Di Huang Wan, a modified version of Liu Wei Di Huang Wan, as it adds two warming herbs, fu zi and gui zhi, to ignite yang qi within the mingmen. This formula is ideal for supporting mutually dependent kidney yin and yang fire and water.

Herbs in the formula: sheng di huang, shan zhu yu, shan yao, fu zi, gui zhi, ze xie, fu ling, mu dan pi.

The primary focus of Jin Gui Shen Qi Wan is to nourish yin and yang, re-inforce blood, tonify the liver and kidney, and preserve essential qi. It has a special ability to support body fluid metabolism and blood circulation. This is especially important in menopausal-transition patients experiencing water retention and circulation issues due to yang deficiency.

Fu zi is added to ignite the source or kidney yang fire. This warms yang qi, dispels cold, and eliminates dampness. Gui zhi is added to warm the channels and unblock the vessels. It also warms kidney yang. By doing so, it warms the bladder and promotes urination to drain body fluid retention.

Jin Gui Shen Qi Wan is normally contraindicated in yin deficiency patterns. It is important for practitioners to diagnose the hot flash properly and decide whether the fire symptoms are actually the result of yin deficiency heat or due to yang deficiency with accumulation of yin fire, in which case, Jin Gui Shen Qi Wan would be appropriate.

YOU GUI WAN

You Gui Wan 右归丸 (Restore the Right Kidney Pill) warms and toni-fies kidney yang, replenishes essence, and tonifies blood. You Gui Wan addresses cases of kidney yang deficiency with decline of mingmen fire. Unlike Jin Gui Shen Qi Wan, it focuses its efforts on tonification, with less attention paid to draining and sedation.

You Gui Wan and Zuo Gui Wan are kidney nourishing cohorts to "restore" the right (yang) and left (yin) kidney respectively.

Herbs in the formula: fu zi, rou gui, lu jiao jiao, shu di huang, shan zhu yu, shan yao, gou qi zi, tu si zi, du zhong, dang gui.

Fu zi and rou gui warm and tonify kidney yang, while lu jiao jiao replenishes yang and essence and tonifies the marrow. Their functions are enhanced by the addition of tu si zi and du zhong. The rest of the formula nourishes kidney yin and tonifies the liver and spleen to aid in essence and blood production. You Gui Wan is a particularly effective hot-flash formula for a small group of patients presenting with yang deficiency symptoms, including fatigue, urinary incontinence, or body fluids and metabolism issues.

Calming the Spirit Prescriptions

Spirit (shen) calming prescriptions calm the spirit and tranquilize the mind. These formulas are needed in the hot-flash environment to help treat menopausal-transition symptoms such as hot flashes, palpitations, insomnia, irritability, restlessness, vexation, and anxiety.

The spirit can become agitated or disquieted by numerous factors. Excess patterns can harass the spirit, while deficiency patterns will lead to malnourishment of the spirit. Excess and deficiency patterns are the result of imbalances of yin and yang, and qi and blood. Constitutional and lifestyle factors create these imbalances. Some people are predisposed to shen disturbances, while others develop them through life experiences. They are a normal part of life. Physical changes during menopausal transition may initiate or exacerbate spirit disruption.

Calming the spirit takes a two-step approach: one of sedation and one of nourishment. This approach treats both the symptoms and the root causes. Formulas in this category utilize spirit tranquilizing herbs, yang anchoring herbs, fire clearing herbs, qi and blood moving herbs, qi and blood nourishing herbs, yin and yang nourishing herbs, and damp-phlegm drying and draining herbs.

- Tian Ma Gou Teng Yin

- Gui Pi Tang

- Chai Hu Jia Long Gu Mu Li Tang

- Suan Zao Ren Tang

- Tian Wang Bu Xin Dan

- Gan Mai Da Zao Tang.

TIAN MA GOU TENG YIN

Tian Ma Gou Teng Yin 天麻钩藤饮 (Gastrodia and Uncaria Decoction) calms the liver, extinguishes wind, clears heat, invigorates blood, and tonifies the liver and kidney. This is an important formula for ascending liver yang with internal movement of liver wind. This is a very common hot-flash environment pattern.

Menopausal transition and hypertension are similar in nature. It is worth noting that many women experience a slight increase in blood pressure once reaching menopausal transition. Tian Ma Gou Teng Yin is well-suited to hypertension symptoms such as headaches, dizziness, vertigo, tinnitus, vision problems, and insomnia.

Herbs in the formula: tian ma, gou teng, shi jue ming, zhi zi, huang qin, yi mu cao, niu xi, du zhong, sang ji sheng, ye jiao teng, fu shen.

The first set of herbs, tian ma, gou teng, and shi jue ming, calms the liver and anchors ascending yang qi and liver fire. This is important to stop excess liver yang, wind, and fire from harassing the heart and shen.

The second set of herbs, zhi zi and huang qin, clears heat and drains fire. They provide additional prevention against heat rising up from the liver and agitating the heart fire.

The third set of herbs targets the blood. Yi mu cao specifically invigorates blood to support proper circulation. It prevents blood from rising to the head along with the ascending yang. Niu xi further aids this by conducting blood downward with its descending action.

The fourth set of herbs, du zhong and sang ji sheng, tonifies and nourishes the liver and kidney. This supports healthy yin and yang for the heart and spirit.

The final set of herbs, ye jiao teng and fu shen, is added to calm the spirit and steady the will.

I have seen more amazing clinical results from using Tian Ma Gou Teng Yin in treating hot flashes than any other formula. I believe it is because of its strong yang and fire sedating actions. It is easy to combine this formula with other appropriate formulas to enhance the kidney and liver yin and blood nourishing effects. I have successfully used Tian Ma Gou Teng Yin to reduce and control tamoxifen-induced hot flashes.

GUI PI TANG

Gui Pi Tang 归脾汤 (Restore the Spleen Decoction) augments the qi, tonifies blood, strengthens the spleen, and nourishes the heart. It is known for its ability to treat insomnia and anxiety due to heart and spleen qi and blood deficiency patterns from overthinking, excessive worry, and rumination.

Herbs in the formula: ren shen, huang qi, bai zhu, zhi gan cao, dang gui, long yan rou, suan zao ren, fu shen, zhi yuan zhi, mu xiang, sheng jiang, da zao.

Gui Pi Tang has two primary sets of herbs. The first set, consisting of ren shen, huang qi, bai zhu, zhi gan cao, and dang gui, carries out the functions of tonifying qi and blood to support the spirit. Nourishing qi and blood roots the spirit.

The second set, consisting of long yan rou, suan zao ren, fu shen, and zhi yuan zhi, calms the spirit. Mu xiang, sheng jiang, and da zao act as assistants and regulate qi and revive the spleen.

Gui Pi Tang works very well at quelling hot flashes in qi and blood deficiency patterns. Si Wu Tang does have a stronger effect on nourishing blood. It is often useful to modify or combine the two formulas to enhance the blood nourishing effects, especially when treating insomnia and anxiety.

Though both Gui Pi Tang and Bu Zhong Yi Qi Tang are effective in treating hot flashes, Gui Pi Tang is often more appropriate, since qi and blood deficiency is slightly more common during menopausal transition than qi and yang deficiency.

CHAI HU JIA LONG GU MU LI TANG

Chai Hu Jia Long Gu Mu Li Tang 柴胡加龙骨牡蛎汤 (Bupleurum Plus Dragon Bone and Oyster Shell Decoction) is a Xiao Chai Hu Tang formula modification. It is used for treating stubborn menopausal-transition symptoms with an underlying pattern of qi stagnation and heat repletion.

Herbs in the formula: chai hu, huang qin, ban xia, ren shen, sheng jiang, gui zhi, fu ling, long gu, mu li, da huang, da zao, qian dan.

Chai Hu Jia Long Gu Mu Li Tang is similar in nature to Xiao Chai Hu Tang, but it goes a few steps further. It incorporates the use of long gu and mu li, a powerful combination to calm the liver, anchor ascending yang, and calm the spirit. It also uses da huang for its effects of draining internal heat.

Chai Hu Jia Long Gu Mu Li Tang is effective in relieving severe hot flashes, insomnia, depression, anxiety, and neurosis in cases of severe qi stagnation and heat repletion that are unresponsive to other treatments.

SUAN ZAO REN TANG

Suan Zao Ren Tang 酸枣仁汤 (Sour Jujube Decoction) nourishes blood, calms the spirit, clears heat, and eliminates irritability. It is suited to cases of liver blood deficiency with deficiency heat. By enriching and nourishing the liver blood at the source, it raises yin and supports the heart. Suan Zao Ren Tang is regularly used as an insomnia formula.

Herbs in the formula: suan zao ren, chuan xiong, fu ling, zhi mu, zhi gan cao.

The chief herb, suan zao ren, nourishes liver blood and calms the heart spirit. Chuan xiong regulates liver blood by encouraging it to flow freely. This combination of one astringent and one dispersing herb nourishes and regulates the liver while calming the spirit.

Fu ling is added for its spirit calming ability and to tonify the spleen and stomach. Zhi mu enriches yin and clears any excess or deficiency heat. It also moistens and protects from the drying nature of chuan xiong. Zhi gan cao regulates and harmonizes.

This is a classic "mother (liver) cannot nourish the child (heart)" scenario. Liver blood and heat from deficiency is a familiar hot-flash environment pattern. Symptoms specific to this pattern include deficient irritability, inability to sleep, palpitations, night sweats, a dry and red tongue, dizziness, and a wiry and thin or rapid pulse.

Suan Zao Ren Tang is a short and elegant formula that can be used alone or in conjunction with other formulas.

TIAN WANG BU XIN DAN
Tian Wang Bu Xin Dan 天王补心丹 (Emperor of Heaven's Special Pill to Tonify the Heart) enriches yin, nourishes blood, tonifies the heart, and calms the spirit. This treats a heart and kidney yin and blood deficiency with deficiency heat pattern.

Herbs in the formula: sheng si huang, dan shen, dang gui, bai zi ren, yuan zhi, ren shen, fu ling, tian men dong, mai men dong, xuan shen, wu wei zi, suan zao ren, jie geng, zhu sha.

Sheng di huang tonifies yin and blood, cools blood, and supports kidney water to abate heart fire. Tian men dong, mai men dong, and xuan shen further nourish yin to clear deficiency fire. Dan shen and dang gui tonify blood and nourish the heart without causing stasis. Ren shen and fu ling support the heart qi to calm the spirit. Wu wei zi and suan zao ren prevent leakage of heart qi to calm the spirit. Bai zi ren, yuan zhi, and zhu sha nourish the heart and calm the spirit. Jie geng conducts the effects of the other herbs upward into the upper jiao.

Focusing primarily on the heart in the upper jiao, Tian Wang Bu Xin Dan works well to reestablish the fire and water balance between the heart and kidney by nourishing yin and quelling heart fire. It is well-suited to chronic hot flashes, especially during late menopausal transition or post-menopause with symptoms including palpitations, anxiety, irritability, insomnia with restless sleep, night sweats, a red tongue with little coating, dry stools, and a thin and rapid pulse.

Gui Pi Tang is close to Tian Wang Bu Xin Dan in that they both treat the heart spirit. The difference is that Gui Pi Tang is better suited to the heart spirit along with spleen qi with qi and blood deficiency symptoms, with pale and weak manifestations, fatigue, poor appetite, and spontaneous sweats.

Both Suan Zao Ren Tang and Tian Wang Bu Xin Dan treat the heart spirit. Suan Zao Ren Tang is better suited to liver blood with deficiency heat issues harassing the heart spirit. Suan Zao Ren Tang is better for early menopausal-transition patients. The key diagnosis is heightened stress, irritability, and a wiry pulse.

GAN MAI DA ZAO TANG

Gan Mai Da Zao Tang 甘麦大枣汤 (Licorice, Wheat, and Jujube Decoction) nourishes the heart, calms the spirit, and harmonizes the middle jiao. It is a classic formula for restless organ disorder or "zang zao syndrome."

Excessive worry, anxiety, or pensiveness injures the heart yin and blood, disrupts the free flow of liver qi, and depletes the spleen qi. Over time, this creates heart blood deficiency, leading to memory issues, uncontrollable emotions, and restless sleep. Chronic emotional stress and blood deficiency causes liver qi stagnation, further disrupting the emotional state. The results are mood swings, irritability, bouts of crying, and sometimes severe issues of hysteria or neurosis.

Herbs in the formula: xiao mai, gan cao, da zao.

Xiao mai and fu xiao mai come from the same plant and are similar in function. Xiao mai is indicated for nourishing the heart and liver to calm the shen, while fu xiao mai is traditionally indicated for treating spontaneous and night sweating disorders. They are interchangeable based on the patient's symptoms. The original formula comes from the Essentials from the Golden Cabinet and calls for xiao mai; many modern patent formulas use xiao mai. Gan cao harmonizes the middle jiao and nourishes the heart. Da zao tonifies the spleen, soothes the liver qi, and nourishes the heart.

Gan Mai Da Zao Tang works well to improve sleep and calm a restless mind. It can be used alone or added to other formulas to reduce common menopausal-transition symptoms.

References

Avis, N. and Coeytaux, R. (2010) 'The role of acupuncture in treating menopausal hot flashes.' *Menopause 17*, 2, 228–230.

Avis, N., Coeytaux, R., Isom, S., *et al.* (2016) 'Acupuncture in Menopause (AIM) study: A pragmatic, randomized controlled trial.' *Menopause 23*, 6, 626–637.

Avis, N., Coeytaux, R., Levine, B., *et al.* (2017) 'Trajectories of response to acupuncture for menopausal vasomotor symptoms: The Acupuncture in Menopause study.' *Menopause 24*, 2, 171–179.

Borud, E. K., Alraek, T., White, A., *et al.* (2009) 'The Acupuncture on Hot Flushes Among Menopausal Women (ACUFLASH) study, a randomized controlled trial.' *Menopause 16*, 3, 484–493.

Chiu, H. Y., Pan, C. H., Shyu, Y. K., *et al.* (2015) 'Effects of acupuncture on menopause-related symptoms and quality of life in women in natural menopause.' *Menopause 22*, 2, 234–244.

Deecher, D. C. and Dorries, K. (2007) 'Understanding the pathophysiology of vasomotor symptoms (hot flushes and night sweats) that occur in perimenopause, menopause, and postmenopause life stages.' *Archives of Women's Mental Health 10*, 6, 247–257.

Ee, C., French, S., Xue, C., *et al.* (2017) 'Acupuncture for menopausal hot flashes: Clinical evidence update and its relevance to decision making.' *Menopause 24*, 8, 980–987.

Flaws, B. (2007) *Li Dong-Yuan's Treatise on the Spleen & Stomach—A Translation of the Pi Wei Lun.* Boulder, CO: Blue Poppy Press.

Freedman, R. R. (2014) 'Menopausal hot flashes: Mechanisms, endocrinology, treatment.' *Journal of Steroid Biochemistry and Molecular Biology 142*, 115–120.

Freeman, E. W., Sammel, M. D., Lin, H., *et al.* (2011) 'Duration of menopausal hot flushes and associated risk factors.' *Obstetrics & Gynecology 117*, 5, 1095–1104.

Fritz, M. and Speroff, L. (2011) *Clinical Gynecologic Endocrinology and Infertility—Eighth Edition.* Philadelphia: Wolters Kluwer—Lippincott Williams & Wilkins.

Halmesmäki, K., Hurskainen, R., Tiitinen, A., *et al.* (2004) 'A randomized controlled trial of hysterectomy or levonorgestrel-releasing intrauterine system in the treatment of menorrhagia-effect on FSH levels and menopausal symptoms.' *Human Reproduction 19*, 2, 378–382.

Harlow, S., Gass, M., Hall, J., *et al.* (2012) 'Executive summary of the Stages of Reproductive Aging Workshop + 10: Addressing the unfinished agenda of staging reproductive aging.' *Menopause 19*, 4, 387–395.

Joffe, H., Guthrie, K. A., Larson, J., *et al.* (2013) 'Relapse of vasomotor symptoms after discontinuation of the SSRI Escitalopram: Results from the MsFLASH research network.' *Menopause 20*, 3, 261–268.

Maclennan, A. H., Broadbent, J. L., Lester, S., *et al.* (2004) 'Oral oestrogen and combined oestrogen/progestogen therapy versus placebo for hot flushes.' *Cochrane Database of Systematic Reviews 4*, CD002978.

Mitchell, C., Ye, F. and Wiseman, N. (1998) *Shang Han Lun—On Cold Damage Translation & Commentaries.* Brookline, MA: Paradigm Publications.

North American Menopause Society (2014) *Menopause Practice—A Clinician's Guide, 5th Edition.* Mayfield Heights, OH: North American Menopause Society.

Pinkerton, J. V. (2012) 'The truth about bioidentical hormone therapy.' *The Female Patient 37*, 16–20.

Romero, S., Li, Q. S., Orlow, I., Gonen, M., Su, H. I. and Mao, J. J. (2020) 'Genetic predictors to acupuncture response for hot flashes: An exploratory study of breast cancer survivors.' *Menopause 27*, 8, 913–917.

Rossouw, J. E., Anderson, G. L., Prentice, R. L., *et al.* (2002) 'Risks and benefits of estrogen plus progestin in healthy postmenopausal women: Principal results from the Women's Health Initiative randomized controlled trial.' *JAMA 288*, 3, 321–333.

Seidman, Y. and Ming, L. H. (2011) *A True Transmission of Chinese Medicine's Principles.* Zheng Qinan Project. Accessed on 26/04/21 at https://gumroad.com/yaronseidman.

Shams, T., Firwana, B., Habib, F., *et al.* (2014) 'SSRIs for hot flashes: A systematic review and meta-analysis of randomized trials.' *Journal of General Internal Medicine 29*, 1, 204–213.

Thurston, R. C. and Joffe, H. (2011) 'Vasomotor symptoms and menopause: Findings from the Study of Women's Health across the Nation.' *Obstetrics and Gynecology Clinics of North America 38*, 3, 489–501.

Unschuld, P. (2016a) *Huang Di Nei Jing Ling Shu—The Ancient Classic on Needle Therapy.* Oakland, CA: University of California Press.

Unschuld, P. (2016b) *Nan Jing—The Classic of Difficult Issues.* Oakland, CA: University of California Press.

Unschuld, P. and Tessenow, H. (2011) *Huang Di Nei Jing Su Wen—An Annotated Translation of Huang Di's Inner Classic—Basic Questions.* Berkeley and Los Angeles, CA: University of California Press.

Wang, R. (2012) *Yinyang—The Way of Heaven and Earth in Chinese Thought and Culture.* New York: Cambridge University Press.

Wiseman, N. and Ye, F. (1998) *A Practical Dictionary of Chinese Medicine—Second Edition.* Brookline, MA: Paradigm Publications.

Wu, X. P., Zhang, S. R. and Jin, L. X. (2006) *Modern Acupuncture and Moxibustion Treatment Success Compendium* 现代针灸治疗大成. Beijing: Chinese Medicine Science and Technology Publishing Society.

Yang, S. Z. and Liu, D. W. (2010) *Fu Qing-zhu's Gynecology.* Boulder, CO: Blue Poppy Press, Inc.

Ziv-Gal, A., Smith, R. L., Gallicchio, L., *et al.* (2017) 'The Midlife Women's Health Study—A study protocol of a longitudinal prospective study on predictors of menopausal hot flashes.' *Women's Midlife Health 3,* 4.

Further Reading

Bensky, D. and Barolet, R. (1990) *Chinese Herbal Medicine—Formulas & Strategies.* Seattle: Eastland Press.

Bensky, D. and Gamble, A. (1993) *Chinese Herbal Medicine—Materia Medica, Revised Edition.* Seattle: Eastland Press.

Blalack, J. (2003) *Yinfire and its Pathomechanism.* Accessed on 26/05/21 at www.chinesemedicinedoc.com/wp-content/uploads/2014/11/Yinfire-EssayII.pdf.

Chace, C. and Shima, M. (2010) *An Exposition on the Eight Extraordinary Vessels—Acupuncture, Alchemy & Herbal Medicine.* Seattle: Eastland Press.

Chen, J. and Chen, T. (2012) *Chinese Medical Herbology and Pharmacology.* City of Industry, CA: Art of Medicine Press.

Chen, J. and Chen, T. (2015) *Chinese Herbal Formulas and Applications—Pharmacological Effects & Clinical Research.* City of Industry, CA: Art of Medicine Press.

Deadman, P. and Al-Khafaji, M. (2001) *A Manual of Acupuncture.* Hove: Journal of Chinese Medicine Publications.

Keown, D. (2014) *The Spark in the Machine.* London: Singing Dragon.

Liu, G. (2015) *Foundations of Theory for Ancient Chinese Medicine—Shang Han Lun and Contemporary Medical Texts.* London and Philadelphia: Singing Dragon.

Lyttleton, J. (2013) *Treatment of Infertility with Chinese Medicine.* Edinburgh: Churchill Livingstone.

Maciocia, G. (1998) *Obstetrics and Gynecology in Chinese Medicine.* New York: Churchill Livingstone.

Maciocia, G. (2004) *Diagnosis in Chinese Medicine—A Comprehensive Guide.* New York: Churchill Livingstone.

Mayor, D. (2007) *Electroacupuncture—A Practical Manual and Resource.* Edinburgh: Churchill Livingstone.

Netter, F. (2003) *Atlas of Human Anatomy—Third Edition.* Teterboro, NJ: Icon Learning Systems.

O'Connor, J. and Bensky, D. (1981) *Acupuncture—A Comprehensive Text, Shanghai College of Traditional Medicine.* Seattle: Eastland Press.

Ross, J. (1999) *Acupuncture Point Combinations—The Key to Clinical Success.* Edinburgh: Churchill Livingstone.

Yang, S. Z. (2020) *The Pulse Classic—A Translation of the Mai Jing by Wang Shu-he.* Portland, OR: Blue Poppy Press.

Yang, S. Z. and Chace, C. (2016) *The Systematic Classic of Acupuncture & Moxibustion by Huang-fu Mi.* Boulder, CO: Blue Poppy Press.

About the Author

Dr. Brian Grosam began his journey into Chinese medicine following the lead of his wife, Pamela, an expert in Shiatsu Anma Therapy and Tuina for over 25 years. During the early years, Pamela transformed their family's lifestyle and health by implementing concepts and modifications based on wellness. Brian was intrigued and began to research Chinese medicine. Interest rapidly became enthusiasm and he enrolled in the American Academy of Acupuncture and Oriental Medicine (AAAOM) in Minnesota.

Dr. Grosam found he had a natural affinity for acupuncture and Chinese medicine. Upon completion of his Master's degree in Chinese medicine in 2005, he realized that the more he learned, the more he wanted to know. It became clear that if he was committed to his studies, he needed to pursue his PhD in China. Pamela, being an adventurist soul, agreed, so they packed up their belongings, sold their house and cars, and moved with their two young sons to China.

They lived and worked in Jinan, China, for nearly three years. As a family, these were some of the most difficult and most rewarding experiences of their lives. Dr. Grosam worked in the Shandong University of Traditional Chinese Medicine (SDUTCM) teaching hospital during the daytime and attended Chinese language classes at night. The hospital was like a busy beehive in which he studied and practiced acupuncture, gynecology, and neurology. China was magical and the family bonded through the experience. They studied and worked hard, but also made time to travel and visited many historical sites in China.

Dr. Grosam earned his PhD in Acupuncture in 2009. His

dissertation was on the effects of acupuncture treatment of menopausal symptoms. Returning to Minnesota, he became a professor at AAAOM, where he taught acupuncture for five years. Along with his teaching, Pamela and Brian opened Sun Acupuncture, an acupuncture and Chinese-medicine clinic, in 2010. In the intervening years, he has honed his skills, including treating many women experiencing difficult menopausal-transition symptoms, especially hot flashes.

Dr. Grosam has written several articles and has lectured on hot flashes and menopausal transition at Western and Chinese-medicine symposiums and teaches online continuing education on a range of subjects.

Today, Brian and Pamela partner as general practitioners to treat every person who comes through their clinic door. Together, they utilize every skill and every bit of knowledge they've learned over the years and share their gifts with the public. Brian and Pamela bring outstanding character and integrity to the medical field and to their community.

Index

acquired constitution 124–5
active lifestyle 125–6, 159–60
acupuncture
  auricular 261–3
  back treatments 259–61
  calming the shen 250–2
  chest and abdominal points 256–9
  clinical research 217–24
  deficiency-patterns point
      prescription 230–40
  depth of insertion 209–10
  excess-patterns point prescription 240–3
  excess/deficiency patterns and 206
  heat and fire clearing prescription 244–50
  individualized prescriptions 267
  length of treatment 211, 264–5
  multi-step approach to 196–204
  neck points 261
  needle sensitivity 204–6
  needling techniques 208–10
  plum pit qi case study 255–6
  point prescription (overview)
      210, 212–3, 216–7
  for qi and blood regulation 206, 252–6
  quantity/frequency of treat-
      ments 225–7, 264–5
  recovery rates 226–7
  for stagnation 207–8
  standardized prescriptions 268
  success rates 227–8
  tidal heat effusion patterns 213–5
  time of day and 211–2, 213–5
  treatment schedule 228–9
  yin and yang balance and 196, 207

acupuncture points
  BL10 (Tian Zhu) 261
  BL13 (Fei Shu) 260
  BL15 (heart) 259, 260
  BL18 (Gan Shu) 260
  BL20 (Pi Shu) 260
  BL23 (kidney) 65, 259, 260
  BL52 (Zhishi) 65
  BL60 (Kunlun) 261
  DU4 (Mingmen) 261
  DU14 (Dazhui) 260
  DU16 (Fengfu) 261
  DU20 (Baihui) 238–9
  DU24 (Shenting) 239–40
  GB13 (Benshen) 252
  GB20 (Feng Chi) 261
  GB26 (Daimai) 258
  GB34 (Yanglingquan) 241–2, 252–3,
    261
  GB43 (Xiaxi) 247
  HT6 (Yinxi) 245–6
  HT7 (Shenmen) 237, 261
  HT8 (Shaofu) 245–6
  KI1 (Yongquan) 65, 251
  KI2 (Rangu) 244–5
  KI3 (Taixi) 65, 234–5, 261
  KI6 (Zhaohai) 65, 244–5
  LI4 (Hegu) 237–8
  LI11 (Quchi) 247–8
  LR2 (Xingjian) 247
  LR3 (Taichong) 235–6
  LR13 (Zhangmen) 254–5
  LU1 (Zhongfu) 257
  LU6 (Kongzui) 255

acupuncture points *cont.*
  LU10 (Yuji) 249
  PC3 (Quze) 250
  PC6 (Neiguan) 242–3, 261
  PC8 (Laogong) 246–7
  RN4 (Guanyuan) 65, 232
  RN6 (Qihai) 231–2
  RN9 (Shuifen) 257–8
  RN10 (Xiawan) 257
  RN12 (Zhongwan) 257
  RN14 (Juque) 257
  RN17 (Shanzhong) 256
  Sishencong (M-HN-1) 252
  SJ5 (Waiguan) 248–9
  SJ6 (Zhigou) 252–3
  SP6 (Sanyinjiao) 65, 233–4, 261
  SP9 (Yinlingquan) 241
  SP10 (Xuehai) 249–50
  SP15 (Daheng) 258
  ST9 (Renying) 258–9, 261
  ST25 (Tianshu) 258
  ST30 (Qichong) 258
  ST36 (Zusanli) 232–3, 253–4
  ST37 (Shangjuxu) 253–4
  ST39 (Xiajuxu) 253–4
  ST40 (Fenglong) 254
  ST44 (Neiting) 242
  Yintang (M-HN-3) 252
alcohol 163
allergies 158
auricular acupuncture 261–3
Avis, N. 111, 264, 265
axis
  HPO 102–5
  lung-spleen-kidney 134

beta endorphin 110–2
bioidentical hormone therapy (BHT)
    117–8
bladder problems 179–80
blood
  formation of 48–9
  progressive loss of 30, 46
  quality of 52–3, 101
  spirit and 49
  yin and yang components of 49–50
  yin and yang dynamics within 50–2
blood deficiency with blood stasis 217
blood stasis 215, 217
blood-pressure medications 189–91

Borud, E. K. 111, 117, 264
brain
  and kidney 70–1
  neuroregulation of 110
breath dynamics 45, 80, 150–4, 200–2
bursts of qi 23–4, 54

channels (six jing) 46–7
chao re *see* tidal heat effusion
chemotherapy 119–20
Chinese medicine theory
  Nan Jing 79–83
  pathophysiology in 100–1
  Pi Wei Lun 84–8
  Shang Han Lun 74–9
Chiu, H. Y. 264
chong mai (sea of blood) 46
chronic diseases 158
circadian clock 148–50
clinical research study 217–24
Coeytaux, R. 111, 264
cold extremities 155–6
complexity of causes 22
congenital constitution 123–4
constipation 76, 199–200
constipation formula 74
constitution
  acquired 124–5
  congenital 123–4
contraceptives 115
current treatments 157–8

damp-evil obstruction 215
damp-heat 87
damp-phlegm (chronic) 204
damp-phlegm stagnation (point
    prescriptions) 216
Deecher, D. C. 109
defensive qi *see* wei qi
deficiency (overview) 38–9, 202
depression 176
diagnosis
  of the breath 153
  of constitution 123–5
  effectiveness of 122–3
  of the hot flash 167–73
  initial 197
  of menopausal-transition
      symptoms 173–81

pattern differentiation and 265–6
pulse 184–5
of temperature tolerance 154–6
tongue 182–3
diaphragm 151–2
diet/nutrition 52, 69, 84, 87, 126, 160–2
digestive regulation 198–9
disease (infectious/chronic) 158
Dorries, K. 109
duration of hot flashes 141

eating habits 52, 69, 84, 87
Ee, C. 268
Eleventh Difficult Issue 80–3
emotional imbalances 127,
    176–7, 202–4, 222–3
estrogen 106–7, 108–10
evidence-based practice 263–8
excess (definition) 38–9
excesses (six) 37
exercise habits 125–6, 159–60
exhalation 45
extremities (cold) 155–6

family history 167
fire
    deficient 90–1
    heart relationship to 66–7
    heat and 34–40
    ministerial fire 36, 43, 84–8
    pathogenic 37–40
    sovereign fire 36, 43
    and water balance 43–4, 151
    water over 44–5
Fire Spirit School 88–91
Flaws, B. 84
foods 52, 69, 84, 87, 126, 160–2
Freedman, R. R. 109, 111
Freeman, E. W. 265
frequency
    of acupuncture treatments 225–7,
        264–5
    of hot flashes 138
Fritz, M. 108
FSH 108
Fu Qing Zhu gynecology 91–7

GnRH 108, 110–2

Halmesmäki, K. 119
Harlow, S. 113
health intake *see* intake interview
heart
    and joy/purpose 127
    kidney and the 65–6
    as monarch of the body 66–7
    relationship to fire 66–7
heart palpitations 222
heart and spleen deficiency (point
        prescriptions) 216
heart symptoms 174
heat
    and fire 34–40
    pathogenic 37–40
    treating (overview) 202
herbal medicine
    blood cooling herbs 274
    blood stasis tidal heat effusion 277
    Bu Zhong Yi qi Tang (tonify the
        middle and augment the qi
        decoction) 277, 298–9
    calming the spirit prescriptions 310–6
    Chai Hu Jia Long Gu Mu Li Tang
        (bupleurum plus dragon bone
        and oyster shell decoction) 313
    Da Bu yin Wan (great tonify
        the yin pill) 305
    Da Cheng qi Tang (major order
        qi decoction) 276, 288–9
    damp-evil obstruction tidal
        heat effusion 277
    dampness drying herbs 273
    Dang Gui Bu Xue Tang (tangkuei
        decoction to tonify the blood) 301
    Dang Gui Liu Huang Tang (dang gui
        six yellow decoction) 280–1
    Dao Chi San (guide out the
        red powder) 281
    deficiency heat clearing herbs 274–5
    diagnostic accuracy and 272
    Er Chen Tang (two cured
        decoction) 295–6
    Er Xian Tang (two immortal
        decoction) 306–7
    Er Zhi Wan (two ultimate pill) 305
    excess heat and fire prescriptions 278–86
    fire purging herbs 272–3
    Gan Mai Da Zao Tang (licorice, wheat,
        and jujube decoction) 315–6

herbal medicine *cont.*
  Gui Pi Tang (restore the spleen decoction) 312–3
  heat clearing herbs 272–5
  Huang Lian Jie Du Tang (coptis decoction to relieve toxicity) 279–80
  Huo Xiang Zheng qi San (agastache powder to rectify the qi) 293–4
  Jia Jian Si Wu Tang (modified four herb decoction) 93
  Jin Gui Shen qi Wan (kidney qi pill from the golden cabinet) 309
  Liang Di Tang (rehmannia and lycium root bark decoction) 92
  Liu Wei Di Huang Wan (six ingredient rehmannia pill) 65
  Long Dan Xie Gan Tang (gentianae longdancao decoction to drain the liver) 284
  patent formulas 271–2
  qi and blood deficiency prescriptions 297–301
  qi stagnation with yin deficiency (case study) 292
  Qing Gu San (cool the bones powder) 276
  Qing Hao Bie Jia Tang (artemisia annua and soft-shelled turtle shell decoction) 307
  Qing Jing San (clear the menses powder) 92
  Qing Shu Yi qi Tang (clear summer-heat and augment the qi decoction) 285–6
  Qing Shu Yi qi Tang (wang shi's clear summer-heat and augment the qi decoction) 277
  repletion and stagnation prescriptions 286–96
  safety 275–6
  Si Wu Tang (four herb decoction) 300
  spleen and stomach qi deficiency tidal heat effusion 277
  Suan Zao Ren Tang (sour jujube decoction) 313–4
  "three yellow" herbs 273
  Tian Ma Gou Teng yin (gastrodia and uncaria decoction) 311–2
  Tian Wang Bu Xin Dan (emperor of heaven's special pill to tonify the heart) 314–5
  tidal heat effusion formulas 276–7
  toxin eliminating herbs 274
  treatment principles 269–70
  Wen Dan Tang (warm the gallbladder decoction) 296
  Xi Fen An Tai Tang (quench the conflagration and calm the fetus decoction) 94
  Xiao Chai Hu Tang (minor bupleurum decoction) 289–90
  Xiao Yao San (rambling powder) 290–2
  Xie Huang San (drain the yellow powder) 282–3
  Xue Fu Zhu Yu Tang (drive out stasis in the mansion of blood decoction) 277, 294–5
  yang deficiency prescriptions 308–10
  yangming excess tidal heat effusion 276
  Yi Guan Jian (linking decoction) 306
  Yi Huang Tang (change yellow (discharge) decoction) 96
  yin deficiency and blood depletion tidal heat effusion 276
  yin deficiency prescriptions 302–8
  You Gui Wan (restore the right kidney pill) 309–10
  Yu Nu Jian (jade woman decoction) 283–4
  Zhi Bai Di Huang Wan (anemarrhena phellodendron and rehmannia pill) 303–4
  Zhi Han San (stop sweating powder) 97
  Zhu Ye Shi Gao Tang (lophatherus and gypsum decoction) 282
  Zhuan Qi Tang (change the qi decoction) 95
  Zuo Gui Wan (restore the left (kidney) pill) 304
holistic approach 22–3, 26–7
hormones
  beta endorphin 110–2
  bioidentical hormone therapy (BHT) 117–8
  during menstrual cycle 105–6
  estrogen 106–7, 108–10
  FSH 108
  GnRH 108, 110–2

HT 116–8
inhibin 107–8
LH 108
norepinephrine 110–2
progesterone 107
hot flashes
  categories of 225
  diagnosis of 167–73
  duration of 141
  frequency of 138
  severity of 139–41
  time of day and 138–41, 142, 145–50
HPO axis 102–5
Huangdi Neijing Suwen 27–31
hydration 162–3
hypertension 189–91
hypothalamus 104–5
hysterectomy 119, 185

infectious diseases 158
inhalation 45
inhibin 107–8
intake interview
  family history 167
  health history 157–9
  lifestyle history 159–63
  menstrual cycle history 163–6

Jin, L. X. 216
Joffe, H. 118, 264
joint discomfort 222
joy/purpose in life 127

kidney
  and the brain 70–1
  essence 65
  and the heart 65–6
  and the liver 67
  and the lower jiao 70
  and the lung 69–70
  and the spleen and stomach 68–9
  true yin and yang of 64–5
  and work/rest balance 126–7
kidney decline theory 30–1
kidney yang deficiency (point
  prescriptions) 216
kidney yin deficiency (point
  prescriptions) 216
kidney-heart dynamics 43–4

kidney-liver-heart trajectory 135
kidney-liver-spleen triad 137
kidney-lung disconnection 80–3
kidney-lung-heart trajectory 135–6
kidney-spleen-heart trajectory 135

large intestine (and digestive regulation)
  199
leucorrhea 96
levothyroxine 187–8
LH 108
lifestyle factors 25–6, 52–3,
  69, 125–7, 159–63
Liu, D. W. 91, 92, 93, 94, 95, 96, 97
liver
  kidney and the 67
  and stress/emotions 127
liver depression 86–7, 216
liver-spleen-heart triad 136
lower jiao and kidney 70
lung (and activity/breath) 125
lung and kidney 69–70, 150–4
lung qi stagnation 201–2
lung-kidney disconnection 80–3
lung-spleen-kidney axis 134

Maclennan, A. H. 117
menopause
  artificial 118–20, 185–6
  premature 100, 118–9
  transition symptoms 100
Menopause Rating Scale (MRS) 173–81
menstrual cycle
  irregularities 164–5, 224
  period symptoms 165–6
  taking history of 163–6
Ming, L. H. 90, 91
ministerial fire 36, 43, 84–8, 203–4
Mitchell, C. 75, 76, 77, 78, 79
mood issues 176–7
muscular discomfort 222

Nan Jing 79–83
night sweating 79
norepinephrine 110–2
North American Menopause
  Society 110, 116
nutrition/diet 52, 69, 84, 87, 126,
  160–2

ovaries 104

pathogenic heat and fire 37–40
pattern differentiation 265–6
penetrating vessel (sea of blood) 46
Pi Wei Lun 84–8
Pinkerton, J. V. 117
pituitary gland 104–5
post-heaven (acquired) constitution 124–5
pre-heaven (congenital) constitution
    123–4
premature menopause 100, 118–9
progesterone 107
pulses
    interplay of 41–2
    pulse diagnosis 184–5
purpose in life 127

qi
    and blood regulation 206, 252–6
    bursts of 23–4, 54
    flows of independent 41–2
qi and blood deficiency 131–2, 297–301
qi regulation (in acupuncture) 197–8
qi stagnation 78, 151–2, 207–8
quality-of-life indicator 226

radiation treatment 119–20
recovery rates (acupuncture) 226–7
relative yin deficiency 128–9, 302
reproductive aging 112–4
research (acupuncture)
    clinical research study 217–24
    evidence-based practice 263–8
Romero, S. 120
Rossouw, J. E. 117

Scroll One 90, 91
sea of blood 46
sea of marrow 70–1
Seidman, Y. 90, 91
selective estrogen-receptor mod-
    ulators (SERMs) 118
seven-year increments 27–31
severity of hot flashes 139–41
sexual problems 178–9
Shams, T. 118
Shang Han Lun 74–9

shen/spirit
    and blood 49
    calming (with acupuncture) 250–2
    treating (for emotional im-
        balances) 202–4
six excesses 37
six jing (channels) 46–7
sleep aids 191–2
sleep problems
    clinical research 221
    evaluating 175
small intestine (and digestive
        regulation) 199
sovereign fire 36, 43
Speroff, L. 108
spirit see shen/spirit
spleen
    and diet/nutrition 126
    and digestive regulation 199
    kidney and the 68–9
spleen qi deficiency 85–6
spleen and stomach deficiency (point
        prescriptions) 214, 216
SSRIs/SNRIs 118
Stages of Reproductive Aging Work-
        shop (STRAW +10) 113–4
stagnations 132–3, 152–3
stomach
    and digestive regulation 198
    kidney and the 68–9
stress/emotional imbalance 127,
        176–7, 202–4, 222–3
success rates (acupuncture) 227–8
sweating 79
Synthroid (levothyroxine) 187–8

"taijitu" symbol 55
Tamoxifen 188–9
temperature tolerance 154–6
ten-women scenario 25–6
Tessenow, H. 28, 30, 49, 145, 272
thermoregulation 102, 154–6
Thurston, R. C. 264
tidal fever 39, 147–8
tidal heat effusion
    at set intervals 75–6
    blood stasis 215
    chao re 31–4
    classifications of 32

damp-evil obstruction 215
from excess heat stagnation pattern 75
herbal formulas for 276–7
spleen and stomach qi deficiency 214
yangming excess 214
yin deficiency and blood depletion 213–4
time of day
for acupuncture 211–2, 213–5
circadian clock 148–50
and hot flashes 138–41, 142, 145–50
of yin and yang cycle 42–4, 142–3, 145–7
tongue diagnosis 182–3
trajectories 134–6
triads 136–7
true yang 64–5, 89–91
true yin 64–5, 89–91, 128–9, 302

Unschuld, P. 28, 30, 49, 60, 80, 122,
        142, 143, 144, 145, 195, 272
urogenital disorders 223–4

vacuity fire and heat 39
vaginal dryness 180–1
variability in women's experience 25–7
"vexing heat" 39

Wang, R. 44
water
    and fire balance 43–4, 151
    over fire 44–5
wei qi
    cycle of 144–5
    as defence 47
    disruption in 60–2
    overview 60
weight 159
Western medicine
    anxiety drugs 191–2
    bioidentical hormone therapy
        (BHT) 117–8
    blood-pressure medications 189–91
    chemotherapy 119–20
    contraceptives 115

ethics/contraindications 115
HT 116–8
hysterectomy 119, 185
multiple medications 157–8
perspective of 21
pharmaceuticals-induced
        hot flashes 186–92
radiation treatment 119–20
selective estrogen-receptor
        modulators (SERMs) 118
SSRIs/SNRIs 118, 191–2
Synthroid (levothyroxine) 187–8
Tamoxifen 188–9
Wiseman, N. 31, 38, 65, 75,
        76, 77, 78, 79, 213
Women's Health Initiative trials 116–7
work/rest balance 126–7
Wu, X. P. 216

yang brightness disease 77
yang brightness patterns 76
yang deficiency 56, 130–1
yang excess 57–8
yang exuberance 129–30
Yang, S. Z. 91, 92, 93, 94, 95, 96, 97
yangming excess 214
Ye, F. 31, 38, 65, 75, 76, 77, 78, 79, 213
yin deficiency 58
yin deficiency and blood depletion 213–4
yin excess 59
yin and yang
    components of the qi 53–5
    cycle of 42–4, 142–3, 145–7
    as diagnostic tool 53–5, 59
    disruption to balance of 54, 143–4
    rise and descent process 55–6
    supporting over time 55
ying qi 47, 49

zangfu organ theory 63–72
Zhang, S. R. 216
Zhi Han San (stop sweating powder) 97
Ziv-Gal, A. 264